1

Addiction Medicine in Primary Care: A Primer for Physicians and Residents

By: James W. Price, Sr., D.O.

Independently Published

Table of Contents

Dedication:

This work is dedicated to my wife Michele and my children, Amanda, Jamie and Aden. Thank you for the sacrifices made while I researched and produced this monograph. You are my inspiration to live a better life.

Chapter 1
Introduction

"There is a principle which is a bar against all information, which is proof against all arguments and which cannot fail to keep a man in everlasting ignorance – that principle is contempt prior to investigation."

- Herbert Spencer

Why should we care about addictions? There are numerous reasons. Addiction affects not only the addict but it also affects everyone with whom the addict comes into contact. Addiction can destroy the addict, their friends and their families. Careers are lost, relationships are broken, and children are left scarred. The economic impact of addiction must not be ignored (Table 1.) (Liese & Chiauzzi, 1995). As healthcare providers, there is much that can be done to minimize the damage and to restore hope. We can help to "take the mess and create a masterpiece" (Fleming, Lawton-Berry, Baier-Manwell, Johnson & London, 1997).

To do this we must first put aside our prejudice and open our minds (Table 2). Old paradigms must be put aside. Chemical dependency has been looked at as a moral issue, as a weakness, as a psychiatric problem, even as demonic possession. These attitudes have created a lack of understanding and tolerance in our society. The addict becomes a pariah. These attitudes are common in the healthcare community and are barriers to helping those in need.

Table 1. Costs of Substance Abuse in Millions of Dollars		
Category	**Alcohol 1995**	**Drugs 1995**
Specialty alcohol & drug services	6,660	5,258
Medical consequences	15,830	6,623
Lost earnings – premature death	34,921	16,247
Lost earnings – illness	77,150	17,481
Lost earnings – crime/victims	7,231	43,829
Crashes fires, criminal justice, etc.	24,752	20,407
Total	166,543	109,832
National Institute of Alcohol Abuse and Alcoholism and the National Institute on Drug Abuse. NIH publication No. 98-4327		

Table 2. Physician attitudes & behaviors associated with a poor treatment outcome.
Negative stereotypes
Competing agendas
Hostility
Pessimism
Excessive confrontation
Low levels of empathy

Addiction is a primary, chronic disease with genetic, psychosocial, and environmental factors influencing its development and manifestations. The disease is often progressive and fatal. It is characterized by impaired control over use of the chemical, preoccupation with the use of the chemical despite adverse consequences, and distortions in thinking, most notable denial. Each of these symptoms may be continuous or periodic. Addiction is manifested by intoxication, withdrawal, and tolerance. **Intoxication** is a reversible substance specific syndrome related to recent ingestion. **Withdrawal** is a substance specific syndrome that develops as a result of cessation of use. **Tolerance** is a need for increasing amounts of a substance to achieve intoxication. **Abuse** is a maladaptive and problematic pattern of use leading to significant impairment. **Dependence** involves tolerance, withdrawal, use of increasing amounts, and a persistent desire for a substance (Liese & Chiauzzi, 1995).

The treatment of addiction has historically followed one of a number of **paradigms**. These paradigms have approached the evaluation and treatment of the addict by using various etiologic models including the biogenic model, the psychogenic model and various moral models. Human beings are more than just their biology or their psyche and so is the addict. The disease of addiction is a complex illness that is either the result of, or cause of, dysfunction in each area of what makes us all human beings. This text will address the disease of addiction using the "Bio-psycho-socio-spiritual model" of illness. As individuals we are the products of our biology, our environment, our socio-cultural backgrounds, our perceptual systems, our behavior, and our spiritual beliefs. If we where to focus on one specific area we would be missing 85 % of the disease of addiction. In subsequent chapters we will try to look at the entire puzzle and put together the pieces in order to try and see the big picture, just as addicts everywhere are trying to courageously put their lives back together.

References:

Liese, B.S., and Chiauzzi, E. (1995). Alcohol and drug abuse. *Home Study Self-Assessment Program.* American Academy of Family Physicians (AAFP) Monograph 189. Kansas City: AAFP.

Fleming MF, Lawton-Berry K, Baier-Manwell, L., Johnson, K. and London, R. (1997). Brief physician advice for problem alcohol drinkers: A randomized controlled trial in community-based primary care practices. *JAMA; 277(13):* pp1039-1045.

Chapter 2
Introductory Neurobiology of Addiction

"Every form of addiction is bad, no matter whether the narcotic be alcohol or morphine or idealism."

- Carl Jung

Since its inception, Narcotics Anonymous has strongly held the belief that all drugs of abuse ultimately affect the individual in the same way. Their book *Narcotics Anonymous* makes this statement. "...We put great emphasis on this, for we know that when we use drugs of any form, or substitute one for another, we release our addiction all over again. Thinking of alcohol as different from other drugs has caused a great many addicts to relapse. Before we came to N.A. many of us viewed alcohol separately, but we cannot afford to be confused about this. Alcohol is a drug. We are people that suffer from the disease of addiction who must abstain from all drugs in order to recover." (Anonymous, 1983). There has been much progress in the study of the neurobiology of addiction since the founding of N.A. This research has confirmed that most, if not all drugs of addiction share a common reward pathway. It appears that differences in this area of the brain are what distinguish the addict from the non-addict.

Imaging:

Positron emission tomography and functional magnetic resonance imaging have provided visual representations of what is happening inside of the addict's head. Acute alcohol and cocaine intoxication has been shown to activate the orbitofrontal cortex, prefrontal cortex, anterior cingulated, extended amygdala and ventral striatum. This is accompanied by elevated dopamine availability. Acute and chronic withdrawal with result in the opposite effect with decreased activation of the above areas as well as decreased dopamine activity. Cue-induced reinstatement or craving appears to involve the reactivation of these areas similar to intoxication. Two potential markers for active substance dependence are decreases in prefrontal cortex activity and decreases in brain dopamine D_2 receptors (Koob, 2006).

Genetic Vulnerability:

Genetic vulnerability to addiction has been identified. Addicts and alcoholics have a higher prevalence of variations of the DRD2 dopamine receptor A1 allele (gene) and cannabinoid receptor (CNR 1) alleles (Blum, Braverman, Dinardo, Wood & Sheridan, 1994; Johnson JP, Muhleman D, MacMurray J, Gade R, Verde R, Ask M, Kelley J & Comings DE., 1997). The finding correlates with a decreased density of dopamine receptors in the reward pathway. The result of this characteristic is an inability to experience the "natural pleasures" from life. The resulting elevation of dopamine that comes with using will flood these receptors. This "unnatural" experience leaves the addict with a sensation of pleasure or euphoria. These genetic findings correlate with decreased amplitude of the P300 component of the event-related potential on electro-encephalographic examination. The P300 wave reflects attention resource allocation and active memory. There appears to be an association between the dopaminergic system and the P300 wave.

A Leu7Pro polymorphism of the neuropeptide Y gene correlates with increased alcohol consumption (Carmí & Farré, 2003). A single-nucleotide polymorphism of the μ opioid receptor gene correlates with increased likelihood of opiate abuse (Carmí & Farré, 2003). A single-nucleotide polymorphism of the fatty acid amide hydrolase gene in associated with increased use of illegal drugs and alcohol (Carmí & Farré, 2003).

Reward Circuit:

Symptoms of addiction include tolerance and withdrawal, which mark physical dependence. Addicts also experience a loss of control over usage despite negative consequences of their actions. They begin to "live to use and use to live". The drive for their usage appears to originate in the **mesocorticolimbic dopamine system**. The system has a positive and negative re-enforcement role. This "reward circuit" originates in the ventral tegmental area, which contains the dopaminergic cell bodies and extends to the limbic structures, including the nucleus accumbens, amygdala and hippocampus. This is the mesolimbic subcircuit. The ventral tegmental area to nucleus accumbens pathways serves as a meter, telling the other brain centers how rewarding an activity is. The amygdala helps assess if an experience is pleasurable or aversive and whether the activity should be repeated. It helps to forge connections between the experience, the generated feelings and other cues. The hippocampus participates in recording the memories of an experience; the associated where, when and who. The frontal region coordinates and processes all of the information to determine the ultimate behavior.

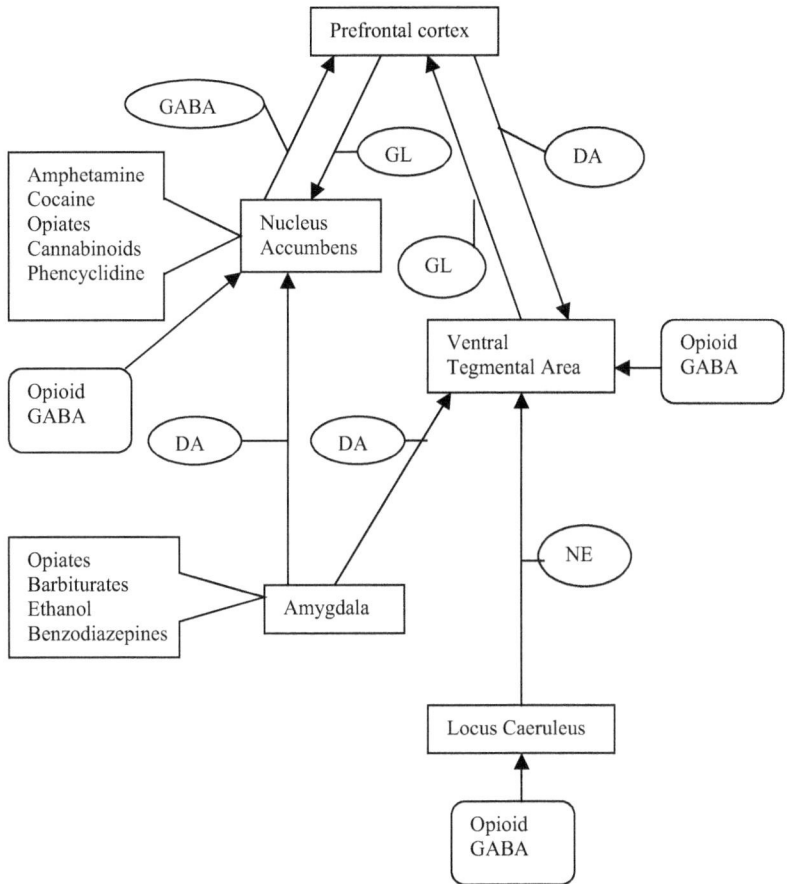

These areas are felt to be involved with the acute reinforcing effects attributed to memory and conditioned responses. Cues related to past drug use trigger powerful emotional and cognitive responses. The drugs of abuse appear utilize the mechanisms of synaptic plasticity associated with reinforcement and reward processing (Kauer & Malenka, 2007). The ventral tegmental area has projects to the olfactory tubercle, the prefrontal cortex, and the anterior cingulate. This is the mesocortical subcircuit. These areas are associated with the conscious experience of drug use, drug cravings and the compulsion to use (Carmí & Farré, 2003). These two circuits work in parallel by way of GABA projections extending from the nucleus accumbens to the ventral tegmental area and prefrontal cortex and glutamatergic projections from the prefrontal cortex to the nucleus accumbens and ventral tegmental area (Carmí & Farré, 2003). These areas are interconnected by the medial forebrain bundle, which contains the monoamine systems (Koob & Nestler, 1997).

Natural pleasures and drugs of abuse, including alcohol, stimulate the release of dopamine from the ventral tegmental area to the nucleus accumbens (Carmí & Farré, 2003). The dopamine responsive cells of the nucleus accumbens increase production of cyclic AMP which activates cAMP response element-binding protein or CREB. CREB is a transcription factor that binds to specific genes triggering the production of proteins including dynorphin which has opium like effects (Nestler & Malenka, 2004). The patient's response is to experience pleasure. As the release of dopamine becomes quicker and more intense the trigger becomes more addictive. The addict will experience **euphoria**, a temporary return to Eden or state of nirvana. Their attempts to become one with the universe ultimately pull them further into Hell. Other neurotransmitters involved in this system are opioid peptide, γ-aminobutyric acid and endocannabinoid (Koob, 2006). Certain drugs have other non-dopamine dependent pathways. These drugs exhibit physical and neuropsychiatric effects that are unique to the particular drug and independent of the reward pathway.

The prefrontal cortex is the region that is responsible for decision making and impulse control. It is not fully developed until approximately after 20 years of age. The earlier an individual begins drinking alcohol and using drugs, the greater the chance they will be afflicted with an addiction. The region will not develop needed connections with other regions of the brain. Defects in this area lead to cognitive difficulties and impulsiveness.

Chronic drug use causes a dysregulation of the reward systems that is marked by a decrease in reward function and limited ability to experience pleasure. Chronic drug use results in sustained activation of CREB and elevated production of dynorphin by neurons in the nucleus accumbens. The neurons loop back to inhibit the ventral tegmental area thus stifling the reward circuit with the induction of tolerance and dependence (Nestler & Malenka, 2004). CREB also play an important role in the transformation of short term memories into long term memories by activating genes that manufacture synapse strengthening proteins (Fields, 2005). The consequence is craving and susceptibility to relapse. This is a common complaint of heroin addicts who are continuously "chasing the dragon" in search of the gratifying response they had with that first high. Serotonergic projections from the raphe nucleus extend to the ventral tegmental area and the nucleus accumbens playing an important role in hedonic mechanisms (Carmí & Farré, 2003). Low levels of serotonin in the nucleus accumbens play a role in the impulsive nature and depressed affect of most addicts and alcoholics after long term use.

Stress or a single dose of any type of addictive substance will activate glutamenergic synapses on dopamine neurons in the ventral tegmental area generating a compulsion to continue using (Carmí & Farré, 2003). Lending credence to the phase, it's the first drink that gets you drunk not the last. The addict is no longer able to experience "natural pleasure" and develops depression. They begin to use their drug of choice just to feel "normal". They seek out anything that will elevate their dopamine levels. Perhaps this is the origin of the expression "sex, drugs, and rock and roll". This dopamine drive becomes the dominant motivator for action in the addict's life, overriding the inhibitory instructions from the cerebral cortex, no matter what the consequences may be. The addict is truly powerless over their addiction (Koob, 2001).

Stress/anti-stress systems:

There is a mechanism in this region of the brain that functions by **negative re-enforcement** involving dysregulation of the limbic-hypothalamic-pituitary-adrenal axis (Goldman & Barr, 2002). It has been hypothesized that elevations of limbic corticotropin releasing factor in the amygdala participates in the mediation of the emotional response to stress and the associated affective changes (Pich, Lorang, Yeganeh, Rodriguez de Fonseca, Raber, Koob & Weissl, 1995). Acute withdrawal of alcohol and other drugs of abuse have been found to cause elevations of extracellular levels of CRF in the amygdala. This may explain the anxiogenic mechanism of withdrawal and act as a motivator for the abstinent addict to use (Weiss & Koob, 1998; Koob, 2006).

Relapse:

The acute abstinent state results in various neurochemical changes that have been implicated in relapse. Decreases in dopaminergic and serotonergic activity have been noted in the nucleus accumbens with drug withdrawal. Increased sensitivity of opioid receptors in the nucleus accumbens is part of opiate withdrawal. Alcohol withdrawal will cause decreased levels of GABA activity and increased glutamate activity (Koob, 2006). Acute withdrawal states may also increase the release of norepinephrine from the locus caeruleus and decrease levels of neuropeptide Y in the amygdala (Koob, 2006).

Compulsive drug seeking behavior is felt to be driven by ventral striatal-ventral pallidal-thalamic-cortical loops (Koob, 2006). This loop involves both the reward pathway and stress system. This is where motivation is transformed into action integrating the reward function and motor functions of the loop. For simplicity the specifics of this process will not be discussed.

The corticostriatal glutamatergic mechanisms of relapse appear to be due to the imbalance between glial and synaptic glutamate release and elimination (Kalivas, 2009). The nucleus accumbens serves as the middle man between the limbic structures and the motor subcircuit. The limbic subcircuit is engaged when a new stimulus in encountered as a means of processing the new information (Kalivas, 2009). This helps the individual determine if they need to adapt their behavior so that they might experience more pleasure or less pain. If the newly established behavior continues to be pleasurable the limbic subcircuit's influence will diminish and the motor subcircuit will become more organized around the task. The limbic subcircuit will re-engage if the behavior fails to yield the intended result allowing for behavioral modification. Addicts experience impairment in their ability to re-engage their limbic subcircuit because of a loss of glutamate homeostasis resulting in compulsive drug seeking behavior despite negative consequences (Kalivas, 2009).

δ-FosB is a transcription factor that gradually increases in the nucleus accumbens with chronic drug use. This molecule is very stable and will persist for months. It engages changes in gene expression that leaves the reward circuit sensitized to drugs of abuse. It is felt that this mechanism leaves the addict prone to relapse (Nestler & Malenka, 2004).

These neuroadaptations may also explain some of the more troublesome changes in behavior that plague the addict. **The LeDoux circuit** is a proposed anatomical basis for the integration of emotions and cognitive activities. LeDoux describes the amygdala as a center for emotional processing and evaluation. The amygdala receives rapid and rudimentarily processed information from the thalamus and the nucleus of the solitary tract. It also receives slower and more processed information from the cerebral cortex (LeDoux, 2000). The above described neurochemical adaptations to drug use would easily affect this region. This may explain the emotional augmentation and poor judgment seen in the individual caught in the chaos of addiction. These changes combined with the consequences of the addict's behavior ultimately create "pitiful incomprehensible de-moralization" and spiritual bankruptcy described by many recovering addicts and alcoholics.

References:

Anonymous. (1983). *Narcotics Anonymous.* Van Nuys, CA: World Services Office, Inc.

Blum K, Braverman ER, Dinardo MJ, Wood RC and Sheridan PJ. (1994). Prolonged P300 latency in a neuropsychiatric population with the D sub2 dopamine A1 allele. *Pharmacogenetics; 4(6)*: pp313-22.

Cami J and Farre M. (2003). Mechanisms of disease: drug addiction. *New England Journal of Medicine; 349(10)*: pp975-986.

Fields, RD. (2005). Making memories stick. *Scientific American; 292(2)*: pp74-81.

Goldman D and Barr C. (2002). Clinical implications of basic research: restoring the addicted brain. *New England Journal of Medicine; 347(11)*: pp843-845.

Johnson JP, Muhleman D, MacMurray J, Gade R, Verde R, Ask M, Kelley J and Comings DE. (1997). Association between the cannabinoid receptor gene and the P300 event-related potential. *Molecular Psychiatry; 2(2):* pp169-71.

Kalivas PW. (2009). The glutamate homeostasis hypothesis of addiction. *Nature Reviews Neuroscience; 10(8)*: pp561-572.

Kauer JA and Malenka RC. (2007). Synaptic plasticity and addiction. *Nature Reviews Neuroscience; 8(11)*: pp844-858.

Koob G. (2006). The neurobiology of addiction: a neuroadaptational view relevant for diagnosis. *Addiction; 101(s1)*: pp23-30.

Koob GF, and Nestler EJ. (1997). The Neurobiology of Addiction. *The Journal of Neuropsychiatry and Clinical Neurosciences; 9(3)*: pp482-497.

Koob GF. (2001). Role of the striatopalidal and extended amygdala systems in drug addiction. *Annals of the New York Academy of Sciences; 877*: pp445-460.

LeDoux, J. (2000). Emotion circuits in the brain. *Annu. Rev. Neurosci.; 23*: pp155–184.

Nestler, E. and Malenka, R. (2004). The addicted brain. *Scientific American; 290(3)*: pp78-85.

Pich EM, Lorang M, Yeganeh M, Rodriguez de Fonseca F, Raber J, Koob GF and Weissl F (1995). Increase of extracellular corticotropin releasing factor – like immunoreactivity levels in the amygdala of awake rats during restraint stress and ethanol withdrawal as measured by microdialysis. *Journal of Neuroscience; 15(8):* pp5439-5447.

Weiss F, and Koob GF (1998). Drug and alcohol addiction: Role of brain CRF systems. *Naunyn Schmiedeberg's Archives of Pharmacology; 358*: R587.

Chapter 3
Alcohol

"First you take a drink, and then the drink takes a drink,
Then the drink takes you."

-F. Scott Fitzgerald

Historically, alcohol was a source of fluid and calories in a time when most water supplies were contaminated. The Babylonians and the Egyptians brewed beer to fuel their armies. The Catholic Church dominated the wine industry for 1300years. These products had much lower alcohol contents than their modern day counter parts. Problems didn't develop until after the advent of distillation by Arab alchemists in 700 A.D. and the production of spirits with much higher alcohol contents (Vallee, 1998).

Ethanol is a simple organic molecule composed of a single hydroxyl group and a short, two-carbon aliphatic chain. The molecule is both lipophilic and hydrophilic making it an amphophile (Hunt, 1990).

Ethanol is a naturally occurring product of sugar oxidation by yeast. This process is termed fermentation. Yeast will die once the ethanol level reaches 12%. This limits the ethanol concentration of fermented beverages. Higher concentrations of ethanol can be achieved by the distillation of the products of fermentation (Hunt, 1990).

Ethanol is almost completely absorbed in the gastrointestinal tract. The rate of absorption is dependent on the amount of ethanol ingested, the rate of consumption, the concentration of ethanol in the beverage, and the presence of food in the stomach. High fat foods have the greatest effect of retarding absorption of ethanol. Ethanol is rapidly distributed throughout the body's water. Equilibrium is first reached in the areas with the greatest blood flow including the brain, the liver, the lungs, and the kidneys.

Ethanol also rapidly crosses the blood-placental barrier to the fetus in pregnant individuals (Hunt, 1990). The fetus is vulnerable to the effects of alcohol. A single episode of consuming two drinks may lead to the loss of fetal brain cells. These infants have a characteristic facial dysmorphia with short palpebral fissures, a thin upper lip, and a long smooth philtrum. They may have under developed ears and clinodactyly (curving) of the fifth finger as well as other abnormalities. The consequences are lifelong, including cognitive impairment and behavioral difficulties (Wattendorf & Muenke, 2005).

Physiology:

Ethanol is primarily metabolized in the liver by two enzyme systems (figure 1.). The primary system is the **zinc-dependent alcohol dehydrogenase system** (Woods & Perina, 2000).

Figure 1:

Primary Pathway: Ethanol Metabolism

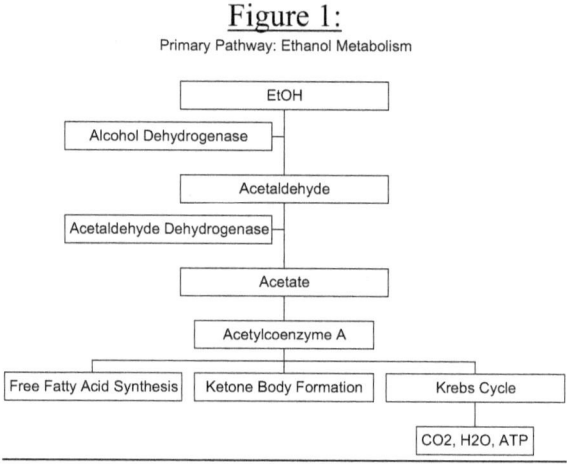

This system metabolizes ethanol at a rate of approximately 10 to 15 ml/hr following zero-order kinetics. The secondary system of ethanol metabolism is the **microsomal ethanol-oxidizing system (MEOS)**. This system is induced by chronic ethanol exposure (Hunt, 1990).

The liver metabolizes 90 to 98% of ethanol. The remainder is excreted unchanged in the urine and expired air. The breath and urine alcohol levels correlate well with the concentration of alcohol in the blood (Hunt, 1990). Law enforcement agencies and alcohol monitoring programs exploit this fact. A patient with a positive breath alcohol should have a confirmatory blood alcohol level (BAL) performed.

Alcohol enhances the activity of the inhibitory neurotransmitter **gamma amino-butyric acid** (GABA); this is mediated by the GABA$_a$ receptor. This initiates a cascade of events, via the endogenous opiate systems, that leads to an elevation of dopamine levels in the reward centers of the brain. The alcoholic is positively re-enforced by these neurochemical changes. Ethanol is a CNS depressant. Initially alcohol will depress the inhibitory pathways of the brain resulting in psychological stimulation and loss of inhibitions. With greater BALs, there will be generalized CNS depression, which will progress to loss of consciousness. Respiratory depression and apnea will occur if the BAL gets extremely high. Ethanol also readily dissolves in neural membranes. Once in the neural membranes, ethanol disrupts the normal movement of sodium and calcium ions, which are responsible for the generation of electrical impulses and the release of neurotransmitters (Hunt, 1990).

Chronic Use:

Chronic ethanol ingestion leads to a number of **physiologic adaptations** (table 1.). One change is diminished functioning of acetaldehyde dehydrogenase. As acetaldehyde builds up, the MEOS will begin to increase its activity. The alcoholic will drink more in order to overcome the effects of the toxic build up of acetaldehyde (negative reward). This physiologic imperative result in a psychological compulsion as the Id's cries convinces the Ego to drink; relying on defense mechanisms such as denial and rationalization.

The mitochondria undergo structural changes that allow them to utilize alcohol preferentially over glucose as an energy source. This helps to support drinking in the early stages, but will later lead to cellular injury or death.

The cells of the brain adapt to chronic ethanol exposure. The cellular membranes undergo structural changes; they eventually weaken and lose stability. The cells will no longer be able to function in a normal fashion. This adaptation is linked to seizures, hallucinations and delirium tremens. **Tolerance** is the first symptom of adaptation. If an alcoholic drinks within their tolerance, their cells will function. If they drink and exceed their tolerance, the cells become overwhelmed and they become **intoxicated**. If the alcoholic stops drinking, the cells go into acute distress as their bodies rely on alcohol as an energy source and to maintain "relative homeostasis" of the neural membranes. This results in the symptoms of **withdrawal** (Milam & Ketchman, 1984).

Table 1. Physiological Adaptations to Chronic Alcohol Use
Diminished acetaldehyde function
Increased MEOS activity
Alcohol becomes preferred energy source
Cellular membrane undergo structural changes
Develop tolerance

Physical Effects:

Chronic ethanol ingestion has other detrimental effects on the body (table 2.). **Alcoholic gastritis** is a disease of diffuse gastric erosions due to chronic alcohol ingestion. This occurs secondary to peripheral vasoconstriction, increased gastric secretions and decreased production of the gastric mucosal protective barrier (Soll, 1996, p 661). **Alcoholic cardiomyopathy** is another disorder of chronic alcohol ingestion. Alcohol and acetaldehyde are direct cardiotoxins. It appears that chronic exposure to alcohol will damage cardiac mitochondria resulting in reversible and irreversible myocardial depression.

The liver is affected by chronic alcohol use (Stevenson, 1996, p 330). **Alcoholic liver disease** encompasses a spectrum of illnesses ranging from fatty liver to cirrhosis. There is increased production and decreased oxidation of fatty acids within the liver. These fat droplets accumulate in the liver causing hepatomegaly and right upper quadrant tenderness. Centrilobular hypoxia occurs with chronic exposure to acetaldehyde. This results in cell injury and death. Hepatocytes metabolizing alcohol will release neutrophil chemoattractants. The recruited neutrophils will release proteases and cytokines causing further tissue damage. The cellular damage results in fibrosis. This will result in alcoholic hepatitis and cirrhosis (Friedman, 1996, pp789-90).

The alcoholic may suffer from **malnutrition** due to decreased consumption of food in favor of alcohol as a caloric source. Decreased absorption of nutrients including vitamins, minerals and amino acids will contribute to malnutrition. Malnutrition will make the alcoholic immunocompromised leading to infections. These malnutritional states may lead to encephalopathy. Confusion, ataxia, abnormal ocular mobility, and polyneuropathy mark **Wernicke's encephalopathy**, which is the result of thiamine deficiency (Hunt, 1990).

Table 2. Physical Effects of Chronic Alcohol Use
Alcoholic gastritis
Alcoholic cardiomyopathy
Alcoholic liver disease
Malnutrition
Encephalopathy

Patients that drink a large quantity of alcohol in the face of relative starvation are at risk for **alcoholic ketoacidosis** (AKA). AKA is a positive anion-gap metabolic acidosis. Starvation decreases glycogen and insulin stores and increases catecholamines, glucagon, growth hormone and cortisol. This stimulates lipolysis and hepatic ketogenesis. Glucose is not available for the Krebs cycle with starvation. The equation shifts to the production of ketone bodies (Figure 1.). Volume contraction is associated with excess alcohol ingestion and will worsen the acidosis. The signs and symptoms of AKA are usually non-specific and the diagnosis should be confirmed by arterial blood gas analysis, serum ketone level and electrolyte levels. Therapy is aimed at glucose and volume replacement. Patients also require thiamine, multiple vitamins and magnesium sulfate (Woods & Perina, 2000).

Withdrawal:

Chronic alcohol ingestion causes a number of cellular adaptations. These changes allow the cells to function in an environment of alcohol and acetaldehyde. The cells are dependent on ethanol for energy, stimulation and sedation. The cells go into acute distress when alcohol consumption is stopped. This results in a life threatening **withdrawal** state. These patients will present with symptoms of anxiety, panic, delusions and hallucinations. They will have signs of psychomotor agitation, hyperarousal, diaphoresis, altered consciousness, hypertension, tachycardia and hyperthermia.

The Clinical Institute Withdrawal Assessment of Alcohol Scale, Revised (CIWA-Ar) uses 10 symptoms and their severity to create a score that can be used to risk stratify a patient withdrawing from alcohol (Table 3.) (Ricks, Replogle & Cook, 2010).

Table 3. CIWA-Ar categories, with the range of scores in each category, areas follow:
Agitation (0-7)
Anxiety (0-7)
Auditory disturbances (0-7)
Clouding of Sensorium (0-4)
Headache (0-7)
Nausea/Vomiting (0-7)
Paroxysmal Sweats (0-7)
Tactile disturbances (0-7)
Tremor (0-7)
Visual disturbances (0-7)

A score of less than 8 is considered mild withdrawal. These patients may be treated as outpatients and most likely need to medications. A score of 8 to 15 is moderate. These patients may require a benzodiazepine but maybe monitored as an outpatient. Score greater than 15 and alcoholics with history of seizures, delirium, suicidal ideation or complicated medical histories require inpatient detoxification with benzodiazepines (Ricks, Replogle & Cook, 2010).

Alcohol withdrawal is treated with a medication that exhibits cross-tolerance with alcohol. Long-acting benzodiazepines such as diazepam and chlordiazepoxide are the agents of choice. Shorter acting benzodiazepines such as lorazepam are indicated for patients with liver disease. These patients need magnesium, thiamine and multiple vitamin supplementations (Milam & Ketchman, 1984; Miller & Gold, 1998).

The abstinent alcoholic will then enter the **"protracted withdrawal syndrome"**. This state is the result of cellular adaptations that have to return to the pre-alcohol state. It takes time for the cells to function normally in an environment that does not include alcohol. This process may take months or years to complete. These patients have to deal with depression, insomnia, agitation, and poor concentration. Negative re-enforcement has taught these patients that alcohol is "the best medicine" for their malady and they may experience strong cravings for alcohol (Milam & Ketchman, 1984).

Pharmacological Therapy:

There have been several **pharmacological agents** used to prevent relapses in alcoholics. Disulfiram was the first medication used for this purpose. Disulfiram interferes with the activity of acetaldehyde dehydrogenase and results in an accumulation of acetaldehyde. The patient experiences flushing, palpitations, and severe nausea and vomiting. Studies have shown that this treatment does not substantially decrease the relapse rate. The selective serotonin re-uptake inhibitors do not decrease the relapse rate except in alcoholics with the co-diagnosis of depression. The most promising agent is the opiate antagonist naltrexone which blocks the μ-opioid receptor leading to reduced dopamine in the nucleus accumbens with alcohol ingestion. The effect of environmental cues and associated alcohol craving can be quelled by pretreatment with the drug. The ideal patient has moderate to severe addiction, has failed prior attempts at quitting and has withdrawn from alcohol. They will need to be withdrawn from opiate if they have a dual addiction and their hepatic enzyme levels should be no greater than four times the normal level. The dose should start at 25mg daily for 1 week then increased to 50mg daily. The medication is best taken with food because of gastric upset and hepatic enzymes should be checked monthly. The usual duration of treatment is 3 to 4 months (Anton, 2008). Both of these agents decrease heavy drinking and relapse rate, but work best in conjunction with cognitive behavioral therapy (Garbutt, West, Carey, Lohr & Crews, 1999; Anton, Moak, Waid, Latham, Malcolm & Dias, 1999).

References:
Anton R. (2008). Clinical therapeutics naltrexone for the management of alcohol dependence. *New England Journal of Medicine; 359(7)*: pp715-721.

Anton R, Moak D, Waid R, Latham P, Malcolm R, and Dias J (1999) Naltrexone and cognitive behavioral therapy for the treatment of outpatient alcoholics: results of a placebo-controlled trial. Am J Psychiatry November; 156:1758-64

Friedman SL. (1996) Cirrhosis of the liver and its major sequelae. In: Bennett JC, Plum F, et al., eds; *Cecil textbook of medicine*. Philadelphia, Pa.

Garbutt JC, West SL, Carey TS, Lohr KN, Crews FT (1999). Pharmacological treatment of alcohol dependence. Areview of the evidence. *JAMA; 281(14):* pp1318-1325.

Hunt WA. (1990). Ethanol and other aliphatic alcohols. In: Craig CR, Stitzel RE, eds., *Modern Pharmacology, 3rd ed.* Boston, Mass., Little, Brown and Co.

Milam JR and Ketchman K. (1984). *Under the influence*. New York. Bantam Books.

Miller NS and Gold MS. (1998). Management of withdrawal syndromes and relapse prevention in drug and alcohol dependence. *Amer Fam Phys; 58(1):* pp139-146.

Ricks J, Replogle W and Cook N. (2010). Management of alcohol withdrawal syndrome. *American Family Physician; 82(4):* pp344-347.

Soll AH. (1996). Gastritis. In: Bennett JC, Plum F, et al., eds; *Cecil textbook of medicine*. Philadelphia, Pa. WB Sanders Co.

Stevenson LW. (1996). Diseases of the myocardium. In: Bennett JC, Plum F, et al., eds; *Cecil textbook of medicine*. Philadelphia, Pa.

Vallee B. (1998). Alcohol in the Western World. *Scientific American; 278(6)*: pp80-85.

Wattendorf D and Muenke M. (2005). Fetal alcohol spectrum disorders. *American Family Physician; 72(2)*: pp279-282, 285.

Woods WA and Perina DG. (2000). Alcoholic ketoacidosis. In: Tintinalli JE, Kelen GD, Stapczynski JS, eds. *Emergency medicine: A comprehensive study guide, 5th ed.* New York. McGraw-Hill.

Chapter 4
Marijuana

"The child without ambition is like a watch with a broken spring."
-R.W. Stockman

Marijuana comes from the leaves of the *Cannabis sativa* plant. This plant was one of the first plants cultivated by humans. It has been used to make fabric, thread, rope and medicines for over 12,000 years. Marijuana is now the most widely used illicit drug in the United States (Cohen, Fleming, Glatter, et al., 1996, pp23-46) The dried leaves and flowers of the plant can be rolled into cigarettes (joints) or put into hollowed out cigars (blunts). Hashish is the processed resin of the marijuana plant that contains a higher concentration of the psychoactive components. Both forms of marijuana may also be eaten, usually in the form of brownies. Dronabinal is the pharmaceutical form of marijuana. It has been used to lower intraocular pressure and reduce nausea associated with chemotherapy.

Pharmacology:

Delta-9-tetrahydrocannabinol (THC) is the primary psychoactive constituent of marijuana. 11-hydroxy-THC, a metabolite of THC also exhibits psychoactive properties. When smoked, the lungs absorb 50% of the THC. Plasma concentrations peak in 10 to 15 minutes with the mind altering effect lasting 2 to 3 hours. Marijuana contains ten times the respiratory irritants, three to five times the tar and carbon monoxide and more carcinogens than tobacco. The GI tract absorbs almost 100% of

THC when eaten. The plasma concentrations peak in 30 to 60 minutes and the effects last 4 to 5 hours (Colasanti, 1990, pp556-558). THC is metabolized through the cytochrome P450 system. One third of THC is eliminated in the urine and two thirds is excreted in the feces (Hollister, 1988). THC has a long half-life and is highly lipid soluble. Marijuana can be identified in the urine 1 to 7 days after a single use and 1 to 4 weeks after chronic use. Ibuprofen, naproxen and fenoprofen may cause false-positive test results (Hals & Richardson, 2001).

Neurochemistry:

There are two endogenous **cannabinoid receptors,** CB 1 and CB 2. The CB1 receptors are G-protein-coupled receptors are primarily found in the brain and are most densely distributed in the hippocampus, cerebral cortex, basal ganglia, hypothalamus and cerebellum. The endocannabinoids, anandamide and 2-arachidonoyl glycerol, are released from postsynaptic cells providing a retrograde signal called depolarization-induced suppression of inhibition (DSI) of presynaptic GABA producing cells temporarily dampening the effects of GABA and enhancing a form of learning called long term potentiation. (Nicoll & Alger, 2004). This process is crucial for extinction or the ability to unlearn conditioned fear (Nicoll & Alger, 2004). There are no CB1 receptors in the respiratory centers. Therefore, THC will not cause respiratory depression. THC also modulates the GABA system. It acts on the CB 1 receptors causing an efflux of dopamine release in the nucleus accumbens and activity in the ventral tegmental area (Carmí & Farré, 2003). THC's action at the CB1 receptors creates euphoria, relaxation, sleepiness, perceived sensory enhancement, and altered time perception. THC has been found to induce neuronal damage and cellular death in the hippocampus. This effect can lead to irreversible memory impairments (Ameri, 1999). The CB2 receptors are found in the periphery. Activity in the areas will cause peripheral vasodilatation and tachycardia (Hubbard, Franco & Onaivi, 1999).

Effects:

THC exhibits a number of untoward physical and neuropsychiatric effects (Table 1 & 2). (Hubbard, Franco & Onaivi, 1999).

Table 1. Physical Effects of Marijuana
Dry mouth
Conjunctival injection
Nausea
Headache
Nystagmus
Tremor
Decreased coordination
Tachycardia
Altered pulmonary status
Altered body temperature
Reduced muscle strength
Decreased cerebral blood flow
Increased food consumption

Table 2. Neuropsychiatric Effects of Marijuana
Anxiety and panic
Paranoia
Confusion
Aggressiveness
Hallucinations
Sedation
Altered libido
Suicidal ideation
Depersonalization
Derealization
Altered perception of time (slowing)
Decline in short term memory
Addictive behaviors

Chronic use of marijuana may lead to impaired pulmonary immune function, which will increase the risk of pulmonary infection. Marijuana is frequently contaminated with Aspergillus, Salmonella and fecal matter further increasing the odds of infection. Chronic abuse of marijuana can adversely affect the cardiovascular system. This is a particular concern in older addicts. Marijuana can cause a dose dependent tachycardia, increase cardiac output, alter blood pressure, increase myocardial demand, decrease myocardial oxygen and increase angina. Marijuana may adversely affect the reproductive system. It can decrease testosterone levels, cause testicular atrophy, cause gynecomastia and change sperm morphology in males. It can reduce fertility, cause menstrual abnormalities and cause birth defects in females. Long-term use of marijuana may result in subtle cognitive defects similar to those seen in aging. Chronic high-dose usage appears to change personality and diminishes interest in personal achievement. This is called **amotivational syndrome** (Hubbard, Franco & Onaivi, 1999).

Tolerance develops slowly. Perceptual and motor functions will be less impaired with heavy use. The subjective effects do not appear to be reduced (Colasanti, 1990, pp556-558). **Withdrawal** symptoms tend to be protracted and subtle because of the high lipid solubility of THC. Patients will be restless irritable and discontent. They may suffer from insomnia and depression resulting from monoamine depletion. Patients may present with nausea, tremor, perspiration, weight loss, and salivation (Hubbard, Franco & Onaivi, 1999). Reassurance and support is usually all that is needed for treatment.

There has been a great deal of debate regarding the safety and legal status of marijuana. Marijuana is not a benign drug. It has the potential to create turmoil in the lives of those that use it and needs to be treated like every other drug of abuse.

References:

Ameri A. (1999). The effects of cannabinoids on the brain. *Progress in Neurobiology;58*: pp315-348.

Carmí J and Farré M, 2003). Mechanisms of disease: drug addiction. *New England Journal of Medicine; 349(10)*: pp975-986.

Cohen G, Fleming NF, Glatter KA, et al. (1996). Epidemiology of substance use. In: Friedman LS, et al., eds. *Source book of substance abuse and addiction*. Baltimore, Md.: Williams & Wilkins.

Colasanti BK. (1990). Contemporary drug abuse. In: Craig CR, Stitzel RE, eds., *Modern pharmacology*, 3rd ed. Boston, Mass.: Little, Brown and Co.

Hals G, and Richardson W. (2001). Drugs of abuse and their complications: Emergency department evaluation and management: Part II. *Emergency medicine reports; 13*: pp147-162.

Hollister LE (1988). Cannabis-1988. *Acta Psychiatr Scand (Suppl) 1988; 345*: pp108-118.

Hubbard JR, Franco SE, and Onaivi ES. (1999). Marijuana: Medical implications. *American Family Physician; 60(9)*: pp 2583-2588.

Nicoll, R and Alger, B (2004). The brain's own marijuana. *Scientific American; 291(6)*: pp68-75.

Chapter 5
Benzodiazepines

"Almost all the ideas we have about being a man or being a
woman are so burdened with pain, anxiety, fear and self-doubt.
For many of us, the confusion around this question is
excruciating."

-Andrew Cohen

Benzodiazepines (BZDs) have been around since the
1960's. They rapidly became the sedative-hypnotic of choice as
they produced less respiratory depression than barbiturates. They
have been used to treat anxiety, insomnia and seizures (Hals &
Richardson, 1999). Prescriptions are the most common source of
benzodiazepines. A substantial amount of the prescribed
medicines are rerouted to illicit sources. Poly-substance abusers
account for 80% of the BZDs abused (Longo & Johnson, 2000).
BZDs are frequently used to augment the effects of other drugs, to
relieve the undesired effects of other drugs, and to relieve the
symptoms of abstinence from other drugs. Flunitrazepam
(Rohypnol®), a BZD, has gained notoriety as a date rape drug
(Hals & Richardson, 1999).

Neurobiology:

BZDs act by causing a conformational change of the
GABA$_a$ receptor. This change increases the affinity for GABA
and activates the BZD-GABA-chloride ionophor complex

resulting in the anxiolytic effects of this class of medication (Longo & Johnson, 2000). This also leads to a cascade of events that result in the stimulation of the central reward pathways of the addict (Koob & Nestler, 1997). Long-term exposure to BZDs causes down regulation of the $GABA_a$ receptor resulting in tolerance to the drug. Loss of the anxiolytic affect occurs in 4 to 6 months (Longo & Johnson, 2000). These medications are metabolized in the liver and excreted by the kidneys. The metabolites can be identified in the urine for a period of 2 to 7 days after the last dose (Hals & Richardson, 1999).

Effects:

BZDs have a number of untoward effects (Table 1.). The most obvious is psychomotor retardation. This results in drowsiness, poor coordination, poor concentration and confusion. These responses will slow reaction time and create a risk for motor vehicle accidents. Patients may also present with diplopia, muscular weakness, ataxia, and vertigo. Large doses may create a state of memory loss similar to the "black outs" associated with alcohol ingestion.

Patients may present with irritability, excitement, hostility, and impulsivity. This is called **paradoxical dysinhibition** and is more common in the very young and very old. Individuals may suffer from emotional blunting and present with depression. This is most likely due to neuroamine depletion. BZDs have been found to be class D teratogens, and intra-uterine exposure can result in fetal dependence and withdrawal (Longo & Johnson, 2000).

Table 1. Effects of BZD Use
Drowsiness
Poor coordination
Poor concentration
Confusion
Diplopia
Weakness
Ataxia
Vertigo
Memory loss
Paradoxical dysinhibition
Depression

Overdose:

BZDs are rarely lethal in overdose, unless they are combined with another sedative-hypnotic like alcohol, barbiturates, neuroleptics, opiates or antihistamines, accentuating respiratory depression. The American Association of Poison Control Centers' 1999 annual report listed 40,000 exposures to BZDs with only 65 deaths. The treatment of overdose is primarily supportive and directed at airway management and respiratory support. Flumazenil (Romazicon®) may be used as a reversal agent, but this medication is generally avoided because of precipitation of acute withdrawal and risk of seizure (Hals & Richardson, 1999).

Withdrawal:

Chronic use of BZDs results in down regulation of the GABA$_a$ receptors and a diminished inhibitory action of GABA. Abrupt **withdrawal** of BZDs creates a rebound of the previously suppressed stimulatory neurotransmitters: serotonin, norepinephrine and dopamine. The patient experiences the symptoms of sympathetic overload (Table 2.). The hallmark is an acute anxiety reaction with elevated blood pressure, tachycardia, tremor and diaphoresis. They may suffer from insomnia and sensory hypersensitivity. The most serious complications of BZD withdrawal are seizures and delirium tremens. Chronic neuroadaptation may cause a syndrome of protracted withdrawal that may last for several months. Symptoms include anxiety, depression, and insomnia (Giannini, 2000).

Table 2. Symptoms of BZD Withdrawal
Acute anxiety
Elevated blood pressure
Tachycardia
Tremor
Diaphoresis
Insomnia
Agitation
Psychosis
Seizures

Detoxification:

Detoxification of BZD addicts is best done in an inpatient setting where heart rate, blood pressure and temperature may be monitored and seizure precautions can be maintained. The goal is to decrease stimulatory neurotransmitter rebound by antagonizing the GABA receptors. BZDs share cross- tolerance with other sedative-hypnotic agents, as they all directly or indirectly act on the GABA receptor. Any of these agents will help to ameliorate the symptoms of withdrawal but a long-acting BZD is the best choice for producing a smooth gradual transition to abstinence. Taper the drug over a period of 6 to 12 weeks if the BZD has been used consistently for several years. Shorter periods of tapering are adequate for patients that use on a less than regular basis or have used the drug for only a few months. The rate of taper is to decrease the dose by 25% at each one-quarter interval of the withdrawal period (Miller & Gold, 1998).

References:

Hals G and Richardson W. (1999). Drugs of abuse and their complications: Emergency department evaluation and management: Part II. *Emergency Medicine Reports; 22(13):* pp147-62.

Longo LP and Johnson B. (2000). Addiction: Part I. Benzodiazepines—Side effects, abuse risk and alternatives. *American Family Physician; 61(7)*: pp2121-2128.

Koob GF and Nestler EJ. (1997). The neurobiology of drug addiction. *J Neuropsychiatry and Clinical Neuroscience; 9(3)*: pp482-497.

Giannini AJ. (2000). An approach to drug abuse, intoxication and withdrawal. *American Family Physician; 61(9):* pp2763-2774.

Miller NS and Gold MS. (1998). Management of withdrawal syndromes and relapse prevention in drug and alcohol dependence. *American Family Physician; 58(1):* pp139-146.

Chapter 6
Opiates

"Thou hast the keys of Paradise, oh, just, subtle, and mighty opium!"

-Thomas De Quincey

Opiates are natural narcotic analgesics that produce morphine like activity. Morphine and codeine are derived directly from *Papaver somniferum*, also known as the poppy plant. Like marijuana, the poppy was one of the first plants cultivated. **Semi-synthetic** opioids are derived from morphine. Heroin was synthesized from morphine in 1874 and became a commercial product in 1898. Heroin became a controlled substance in 1914 under the Harrison Narcotic Act. Hydromorphone (Dilaudid®) and oxycodone (Tylox®, Percocet®) are also semi-synthetics. Purely **synthetic** opioids include meperidine (Demerol®), propoxyphene (Darvocet®), diphenoxylate (Lomotil®), fentanyl, methadone, buprenorphine (Buprenex®), and pentaxocine (Talwin®) (Hals & Richardson, 2001).

Demographics:

Most heroin abusers/addicts are between the ages of 18 to 25 years old. 80% of new users are younger than 26 years old. The purity of heroin has increased in recent years, while the price has decreased. This has increased usage by the middle-class sector of the population, though heroin abuse is still predominately a lower class problem. The present increase in purity has also lead to more deaths secondary to overdose (Hals & Richardson, 2001).

Between 1999 and 2002 oxycodone prescriptions increased 50%, fentanyl prescriptions increased 150% and morphine prescriptions increased 60% with a 91.2% increase in deaths due to opioid toxicity (Compton & Volkow, 2006; Paulozzi, Budnitz & Xi, 2006). The prevalence of prescription drug abuse and dependency in patients receiving legitimate opiate therapy is not insignificant; ranging from 17.8% to 39% (Manchikanti, Pampati, Dammon, et al., 2001; Manchikanti, Pampati, Dammon, et al., 2001b; Manchikanti, Fellows, Darmon, Pampati & McManus, 2005).

Metabolism:

Morphine is greatly affected by **first-pass metabolism**. This reduces the amount of drug reaching the circulation after oral ingestion. Morphine is rapidly distributed throughout the body once it enters the bloodstream. Morphine is metabolized in the **liver** to normorphine. Normorphine and morphine are conjugated as the monoglucurinde or the diglucurinide. These metabolites are then excreted in the **urine** and may be identified by rapid assay. They will be detectable for 1 to 4 days. Dextromethorphan, chlorpromazine and poppy seeds may cause false-positive screening results (Colasanti, 1990).

Neurochemistry:

The reward function of opiates is primarily mediated by the opiates' interaction with **Mu receptors**. These receptors are primarily located in the periaqueductal gray, the medial thalamus, and the nucleus raphe magnus as part of the beta-endorphin system (Colasanti, 1990).Action at this level produces euphoria and analgesia. The **mesocorticolimbic-dopamine system** is involved by indirect activation of GABA inhibitory neurons in the ventral tegmental area, resulting in elevations of dopamine and positive re-enforcement (Koob & Nestler, 1997). These drugs also inhibit the release of norepinephrine in the **locus caeruleus**, which is located in the pons, causing suppression of sympathetic activity (Nistico & Nappi, 1993).

Effects:

Opiates produce a variety of **clinical effects**, including euphoria, analgesia, cough suppression, respiratory depression, sedation, miosis, mild hypotension, decreased gastrointestinal tone, and seizures. **Respiratory depression** is the most troubling of these effects. Opiates blunt the medulla's response to rising levels of arterial carbon dioxide, causing hypoventilation. This occurs prior to the onset of sedation. Hypoxia may cause extreme pulmonary vasoconstriction that damages pulmonary capillaries casing them to leak, resulting in noncardiogenic pulmonary edema (Colasanti, 1990). Miosis or pupillary constriction happens because of opiate interaction with the Edinger-Westphal nucleus of the oculomotor nerve (Hals & Richardson, 2001). Opiate abuse and overdose has no direct cardiotoxic effects. Patients may experience mild hypotension due to histamine release and loss of sympathetic tone to the capacitance vessels of the legs and abdomen (Hals & Richardson, 2001; Colasanti, 1990). Patients that have hypoxic CNS damage may be hypotensive and bradycardic. Opiates depress smooth muscle contractions in the gastrointestinal tract, leaving the patient constipated. Opiates may potentate sphincter of Odi spasm resulting in abdominal pain, similar to biliary colic. Many oral opiate preparations contain acetaminophen. Acetaminophen toxicity may cause irreversible hepatic injury. Seizures may occur because of CNS excitation (Hals & Richardson, 2001).

Abuse:

Addicts that push opiates intravenously have described a warm flushing of the skin and sensations in the lower abdomen that resemble the sensation of an orgasm. This initial feeling is described as a "**rush**". This is followed by a more prolonged sense of euphoria, dominated by feelings of relaxation, contentment, and tranquility. This is termed the "**nod**" (Colasanti, 1990).

Patients that use opiates on a chronic basis will develop **tolerance**. The beta-endorphin system will become functionally deficient with chronic opiate abuse (Giannini, 2000). These patients will have an increased subjective response to pain. Tolerance will rapidly develop to analgesia and euphoria. Tolerance to respiratory depression develops at a slower rate. This places the patient at risk for overdose and hypoventilation as they attempt to gain the same euphoric affects they experienced when they first began using. Little tolerance develops to the stimulant and gastrointestinal effects of these drugs. Patients that exhibit tolerance to one opiate will have cross-tolerance to other narcotic analgesics, but not to other CNS depressants (Colasanti, 1990).

Overdose:

Respiratory depression is the hallmark of opiate **overdose** (table 1.). Other physical signs are miosis, needle tracks, bradycardia, frothy sputum, hypothermia, and coma. Airway management and ventilator support, are the mainstays of treatment. Opiate reversal may also be attempted and should not be withheld for fear of precipitating acute withdrawal. Reversal can be achieved safely by starting with a test dose of naloxone (Narcan®) 0.4 mg IV. If no response is noted, give 2 mg IV every three minutes until the patient responds or reaches a total dose of 10 mg. If the patient responds to the test dose continue to give incremental doses of 0.4 mg IV until the desired clinical effect is observed. Activated charcoal is indicated for oral opiate overdoses. Sorbitol should be included to counteract delayed gastrointestinal motility. These patients will also need to have acetaminophen and acetylsalicylic acid levels drawn as many oral opiates are combined with these compounds and these compounds are toxic themselves (Hals & Richardson, 2001).

Table 1. Opiate Overdose
Respiratory depression
Bradycardia
Pulmonary edema
Hypothermia
Coma

Withdrawal:

The **withdrawal syndrome** associated with opiate dependence is characterized by symptoms that are opposite to the acute effects of opiate use (table 2.). Opiate withdrawal results in hyperactivity in the locus caeruleus, causing a norepinephrine "dump" and sympathetic stimulation (Nistico & Nappi, 1993). This in coupled with corticotropin releasing factor elevations and dopamine depressions result in negative re-enforcement (Koob & Nestler, 1997). These patients present with nausea, diarrhea, coughing, yawning, lacrimation, mydriasis, rhinorrhea, sweating, dysphoria, mild hypertension, tachycardia and drug craving. They may also exhibit piloerection or goose bumps, hence the term "cold turkey". Many patients will have myoclonic leg jerking with muscle cramps. This is the origin of the phrase "kicking the habit". This syndrome is quite uncomfortable but is not life threatening (Hals & Richardson, 2001).

Treatment of opiate withdrawal is supportive in nature. The patient can be made more comfortable by reducing the rate of noradrenergic release with clonidine (Catapress®) 17mcg per kg per day divided into three or four doses. After several days clonidine should be tapered gradually.

Patients may also be given methadone, which is a legal opiate analog that may be used as a substitute and can be gradually withdrawn. Federal regulations do not allow methadone to be used for detoxification if opiate withdrawal is the primary diagnosis. Methadone may be used if the primary diagnosis is a medical condition that required opiate use and resulted in a secondary diagnosis of opiate dependence (Hals & Richardson, 2001).

Ultra rapid opiate detoxification (UROD) is an option for patients that cannot withstand the symptoms of withdrawal. These patients are given a combination of naloxone, naltrexone and clonidine while under general anesthesia. In one study, 55% of 123 patients remained relapse free for six months after undergoing UROD. (Albanese, Gervitz, Oppenheim, Field, Abels & Eustace, 2000).

Table 2. Opiate Withdrawal
Nausea
Diarrhea
Coughing
Yawning
Lacrimation
Mydriasis
Rhinorrhea
Dysphoria
Tachycardia
Cravings
Piloerection
Myoclonic leg jerking

There are several **medications** that improve the abstinence rates in opiate addicts seeking recovery. Methadone has been shown to help retain patients in treatment and to help decrease illegal drug use. It lowers the risk of contracting and transmitting HIV and hepatitis B and C. Candidates for methadone maintenance must have a history of opiate dependence for at least one year and be at least 18 years old. Patients between 16 and 18 years old may be considered if they have been opiate dependent with two unsuccessful detoxification attempts and have parental consent. Methadone maintenance is usually managed by dedicated clinics. These clinics also provide counseling and rehabilitation services. Early induction doses of methadone are used to attenuate withdrawal symptoms and diminish cravings, while preventing euphoria and sedation that will occur with overmedication. The patient should be detoxified once they demonstrate long-term abstinence and possess supportive resources, such as stable income, stable home life and twelve-step involvement (Krambeer, McKnelly, Gabrielli & Penick, 2001).

Naltrexone is a medication with pure opiate antagonist activity. It blocks the opiate receptors and prevents euphoria if the addict succumbs to drug cravings, extinguishing the positive re-enforcing effect of the narcotic (Colasanti, 1990). This medicine should not be used until the patient has been totally detoxified. Naltrexone is usually self administered and can be over ridden by very large doses of narcotics. Therefore, therapy is dependent on patient compliance.

References:
Albanese AP, Gervitz C, Oppenheim B, Field JM, Abels I and Eustace JC. (2000). Outcome and 6 month follow up of patients after ultra rapid opiate detoxification. *Journal of Addiction Disorders;19(2)*: pp11-28.

Colasanti BK. (1990). Narcotic analgesics and antagonists. In: Craig CR, Stitzel RE, eds. *Modern pharmacology*. Boston, Mass. Little, Brown and Co.

Compton, W. and Volkow, N. (2006). Major increases in opioid abuse in the United States: concerns and strategies. *Drug and Alocohol Dependence*; *81:* pp103-107.

Giannini JA. (2000). An approach to drug abuse, intoxication and withdrawal. *American Family Physician; 61(9)*: pp2763-2774.

Hals G and Richardson W (2001). Drugs of abuse and their complications: Emergency department evaluation and management: Part I. *Emergency medicine reports; 12*: pp131-146.

Koob GF and Nestler EJ. (1997). The neurobiology of drug addiction. *J Neuropsychiatry and Clinical Neurosciences; 9(3):* pp482-497.

Krambeer LL, McKnelly WV, Gabrielli W and Penick E. (2001). Methadone therapy for opioid dependence. *American Family Physician; 63(12):* pp2404-2411.

Manchikanti, L., Fellows, B., Darmon, K., Pampati, V. and McManus, C. (2005). Prevalence of illicit drug use among individuals with chronic pain in the commonwealth of

Kentucky: an evaluation of patterns and trends. *Journal of the Kentucky Medical Association*; *103(2):* pp55-62.

Manchikanti. L., Pampati, V. Dammon, K., et al. (2001). Prevalence of opioid abuse in interventional pain medicine practice settings: a randomized clinical evaluation. *Pain Physician*; *4:* pp358-365.

Manchikanti. L., Pampati, V. Dammon, K., et al. (2001b). Prevalence of prescription drug abuse and dependency in patients with chronic pain in western Kentucky. *Journal of the Kentucky Medical Association*; *101:* pp511-517.

Nistico G and Nappi G. (1993). Locus caeruleus, an integrative station involved in the control of several vital functions. *Functional Neurology;* *14*: pp465-488.

Paulozzi, L., Budnitz, D., and Xi, Y. (2006). Increasing deaths from opioid analgesics in the United States. *Pharmacoepidemiology and Drug Safety*; *15:* pp618-627.

Chapter 7
Amphetamines and Related Compounds

The chemistry of dissatisfaction is as the chemistry of some marvelously potent tar. In it are the building stones of explosives, stimulants, poisons, opiates, perfumes and stenches.

-Eric Hoffer

Amphetamine:

Amphetamine was first synthesized in 1887 in Germany. This drug had no clinical use until the 1930's when amphetamine was sold as an inhaler for the treatment of nasal congestion. Amphetamines were used during World War II by Nazi storm troopers for performance enhancement (Narconon, 2011). Amphetamines are currently used for appetite suppression, narcolepsy and attention deficit disorder, but 80% of legally produced pills are diverted for illicit use. Amphetamines are abused for performance enhancement and for getting "high" (Hals & Richardson, 2001). These drugs can be ingested orally, insufflated nasally, or injected intravenously. Injection of crushed tablets has the potential problem of producing talc emboli, which may result in pulmonary emboli or stroke. Amphetamines have several complications associated with their use (Table 1.) (Giannini, 2000). Modern medications used to treat ADHD and obesity, such as methylphenidate and dextroamphetamine, are in this class of drugs having similar issues and abuse potential.

Table 1. Complications of Amphetamine Use
Hypertension
Dysrhythmias
Stroke
Myocardial infarction
Seizure
Tremor
Anorexia
Insomnia
Depression/suicide
Anxiety
Psychosis

Methamphetamine:

Methamphetamine also known as, "speed", "meth", "chalk", "ice", "crank", "crystal", and "glass", was discovered in Japan in 1919. It is easily synthesized from readily available chemicals and is manufactured primarily in clandestine laboratories by using the ephedrine/pseudoephedrine reduction method (Narconon, 2011). This process commonly employs lead acetate as a reagent. Errors in the manufacturing process may create a risk for lead toxicity (Narconon, 2011b). Methamphetamine laboratories are associated with the production of toxic waste, heavy metal contamination and explosions. It may be taken orally, intra-nasally, intravenously, rectally or by smoking. It is most commonly used by white males and is popular in the male homosexual community increasing transmission of

HIV and hepatitis C virus (Winslow, Voorhees & Pehl, 2007). The effects of methamphetamine are similar to the effects of amphetamines but are much more pronounced due to increased potency. Methamphetamine has been a growing problem in the United States since the late 1980's and early 1990's (Methamphetamine Addiction, 2011). There are a number of complications of methamphetamine use (Table 2.) (Hals & Richardson, 2001). **Methcathinone** (Cat) is another designer drug with similar properties. This drug is more popular in Eastern Europe and Russia.

Table 2. Complications of Methamphetamine Use
Hypertension
Stroke
Myocardial infarction
Dysrhythmias
Tremor
Anxiety
Depression/suicide
Pulmonary edema
Psychosis/paranoia
Seizure
Insomnia
Anorexia
Hyperthermia
Lead toxicity

Methamphetamine Derived Club Drugs:

The German company Merck first patented **3,4-methylenedioxymethamphetamine** (MDMA), often called "XTC", "ecstasy", and "Adam", in 1913, to be used as a diet pill. The drug was not marketed for that use. In 1965 Alexander Shulgin, Ph.D. was the first recorded human to use this drug and encouraged research into the use of MDMA to aid psychotherapy. It is currently classified as having no accepted medical use. Illicit use of this drug gained popularity in the late 1980s and it become a schedule I narcotic (Gahlinger, 2004). MDMA is structurally similar to methamphetamine and mescaline, and has amphetamine and hallucinogenic properties making it popular in the "club" and rave scenes (Ecstasy Addiction, 2011). This drug is usually taken orally, but it is occasionally snorted and smoked, but rarely injected. Most MDMA comes from clandestine labs located in Belgium and the Netherlands. It is commonly adulterated with caffeine, dextromethorphan, pseudoephedrine and LSD (Gahlinger, 2004). **3,4-methoxy-N-ethylamphetamine** (MDEA, Eve) and **2,5-dimethoxy-4-methylamphetamine** (STP) are designer drugs with similar properties. These drugs are odorless, tasteless, and colorless and easily transported making them difficult to detect by law enforcement agencies. The unique properties of MDMA create a slightly different spectrum of side effects (Table 3.) (Hals & Richardson, 2001).

Table 3. Complications of MDMA Use
Dysrhythmias
Hyperthermia
Hypertension
Disseminated intravascular coagulopathy
Rhabdomyolysis
Acute renal failure
Stroke
Fulminant hepatic failure: acne like rash is first indication
Seizures
Coma
Bruxism
Sexual dysfunction

Neurochemistry:

Amphetamines enhance the release and block the re-uptake of catecholamines (Giannini, 2000). They may also directly stimulate catecholamine receptors. This accounts for the **sympathomemetic** effects of this drug class including, agitation, tachycardia, hypertension, trauma and insomnia. This yields a rapid release of dopamine in the nucleus accumbens resulting in euphoria (Narconon, 2011b). Some metabolites inhibit monoamine oxidase increasing cytoplasmic concentrations of norepinephrine. MDMA also causes a rapid release of serotonin, accounting for its hallucinogenic properties (Gahlinger, 2004). Amphetamines are readily absorbed after oral ingestion. Several catabolic pathways metabolize it, but a great deal of the drug is excreted unchanged in the **urine**. The drug may remain testable in the urine for up to 2 days. Ephedrine, methylphenidate, phenylpropanolamine, desipramine and amantadine may yield false-positive results. Over-the-counter weight reducing and decongestant products may also create false-positives. Positive tests should be confirmed by gas chromatography and mass spectroscopy (Hals & Richardson, 2001).

Use and Abuse:

Stimulant abusers tend to follow a pattern of binge usage. Addicts that smoke or inject methamphetamine will experience the **"rush"**. This is an intense feeling of euphoria that has been equated to ten orgasms and is very psychologically addictive. The "rush" lasts between 5 and 30 minutes. The **"high"** or the **"shoulder"** follows the "rush". This is the initial response for the addict that ingests or snorts meth. The user feels energetic, aggressively smarter and may become argumentative. The "high" will last 4 to 6 hours. Addicts often try to perpetuate the "high" and to re-experience the "rush". They will do this with the **"binge"** or the **"run"**. Addicts will give themselves repeat doses of the drug, up to 1 gram intravenously every 2 to 3 hours. This can continue for 3 to 15 days, until they run out of drug or become too disorganized to continue. They rapidly develop tolerance to the "rush" and it becomes less intense with each dose. Eventually there will be no "rush" and no "high". Patients at this stage will experience feelings of emptiness and dysphoria. This is referred to as **"tweaking"**. "Tweakers" are very dangerous. Negative re-enforcement makes them crave more meth, but the drug no longer gives the desired response. These individuals experience uncontrollable frustration, resulting in unpredictability and a potential for violence. The stimulant effects of the drug will give those taking it exaggerated movements, disorganized thinking and horizontal-gaze nystagmus. Some addicts will try to ameliorate this problem with a depressant like alcohol or heroin. They will get some symptom relief, but they become a **"disinhibited tweaker"**. They are even more dangerous because of the lack of inhibitions and impulse control. The user experiences the "crash" once they have depleted their catecholamine stores. These individuals become almost lifeless and may sleep for 1 to 3 days. They will also binge eat and become severely depressed or even suicidal. Their bodies will attempt to normalize after the **"crash"**. They will return to a state slightly below their pre-using state as their catecholamine levels are restored (Narconon, 2011b).

 MDMA abuse does not follow the same pattern. Peak plasma levels are reached 2 to 3 hours after ingestion and last between 4 and 6 hours. The user experiences euphoria, verbosity, and sociability along with the stimulant effects. MDMA is known for its enhanced hallucinogenic effects of intense color schemes and sensations. These properties have made the drug popular in the rave setting. The adrenergic properties of the drug allow the patient to dance for extended periods. These individuals will rarely drink enough to maintain an appropriate level of hydration. MDMA may cause hyponatremia by elevating levels of antidiuretic hormone in association with increased water intake. These effects make the abuser vulnerable to seizures. Rapid tolerance develops to the psychoactive properties of this drug, while little tolerance develops to dysphoria, paranoia and anxiety.

This causes the addict to self-limit their usage, and prevents them from "bingeing" (Hals & Richardson, 2001).

MDMA and methamphetamine have both been shown to cause permanent **brain damage**. Methamphetamine has been shown to damage nerve terminals that produce dopamine in the striatum and places the addict at risk for a Parkinson's like syndrome, tardive dyskinesia, and Huntington's chorea (Ernst, Chang, Leonido-Lee, & Speck, 2000). Meth also induces apoptotic neuron death in the frontal cortex, the hippocampus and the striatum. This may leave the addict with impaired memory, cognitive function and decision making capacity (Cadet, Ordonez & Ordonez, 1997). MDMA appears to selectively damage serotonin-producing neurons of the neocortex and the hippocampus. Patients may be left with depression, impaired memory, impaired impulse control, aggressiveness and impaired sleep (Fischer, Hatzidimitriou, Wlos, Katz, & Ricaurte, 1995).

Treatment:

The treatment of amphetamine and amphetamine analog **overdose** is focused on treating the affects of sympathetic over stimulation. **Psychotic** patients should be given benzodiazepines. Refractory cases may be given haloperidol, unless they have overdosed on MDMA. Giving them haloperidol may trigger serotonin syndrome and worsen the psychotic event. Ondansetron, a 5-HT3 (serotonin) receptor antagonist, may help to ameliorate psychotic symptoms. **Seizures** are treated with diazepam and phenytoin if there is no response. Patients with **tachycardia** may be given beta-blockers, but they should be co-administered with alpha-blockers to avoid triggering a hypertensive crisis.

Hypertension can be treated with alpha and beta-blockade, or with nitroprusside. **Hyperthermic** patients need active cooling and urinalysis for evidence of myoglobinuria to rule out rhabdomyolysis. **Myocardial infarction** and **stroke** are possible and managed per ACLS protocol (Perrone & Hoffman, 2000)

      Withdrawal from these drugs poses no acute physical threat. Patients will usually experience social withdrawal, psychomotor retardation, hypersomnia, depression, paranoia and hyperphagia. These symptoms may last for 5 to 7 days. The addict will notice an increase in depression and anhedonia after 30 to 90 days. They will have strong cravings to use that are driven by the depletion of dopamine in the reward pathway. This creates a significant risk of relapse for these individuals. Treatment of this phase of recovery is directed at the symptom of depression and potential for suicide. Bromocriptine, a dopamine agonist, has been used to quell the effects of dopamine depletion. Bromocriptine is started at a dose of 0.625 to 2.5 mg orally three times daily. The drug is then tapered by 0.625 mg per day over the next three to ten days. Desipramine increases the sensitivity of dopamine and norepinephrine receptors. It may help to ameliorate cravings and depression. Desipramine or imipramine may be used alone or with bromocripine. The initial dose is 50 mg daily and titrated upward by 50 mg every other day until a dosage of 150 to 250 mg is reached. This dose is maintained for three to six months and may be tapered off over a period of two weeks (Giannini, 2000; Winslow, Voorhees & Pehl, 2007).

      The Matrix model has demonstrated success in treating those addicted to amphetamines including methamphetamine. This model is an individualized outpatient program using individual, group and family therapy in concert with drug testing and 12-step program participation (Winslow, Voorhees & Pehl, 2007).

References:

Cadet JL, Ordonez SV and Ordonez JV. (1997). Methamphetamine induces apoptosis in immortalized neural cells: Protection by the proto-oncogene, bcl-2. *Synapse; 25:* pp176-184.

Ecstasy Addiction. (2011). *Ecstasy Addiction* Accessed December 9, 2011 from: www.ecstasyaddiction.com/ecstasy-facts/ecstasy-addiction/.

Ernst T, Chang L, Leonido-Lee M and Speck O. (2000). Evidence for long-term neurotoxicity associated with methamphetamine abuse: a 1 H MRS study. *Neurology; 54(6):* pp1344-1349.

Fischer C, Hatzidimitriou G, Wlos J, Katz J, and Ricaurte G. (1995). Reorganization of ascending 5-HT axon projections in animals previously exposed to recreational drug 3,4-methelenedioxymethamphetamine. *Journal of Neuroscience; 15:* pp5476-5485

Gahlinger P. (2004). Club drugs: MDMA, gamma-hydroxybutyrate, rohypnol and ketamine. *American Family Physician; 69(11)*: pp2619-2626.

Giannini JA. (2000). An approach to drug abuse, intoxication and withdrawal. *American Family Physician; 61(9)*: pp2763-2774.

Hals G and Richardson W. (2001). Drugs of abuse and their complications: Emergency department evaluation and management: Part II. *Emergency medicine reports; 22(13)*: pp147-162.

Narconon. (2011). *The history of methamphetamine.* Accessed December 9, 2011 from: www.methamphetamineaddiction.com/methamphetamine _hist.html

Narconon. (2011b). *Methamphetamine information.* Accessed December 9, 2011 from: www.methamphetamineaddiction.com/methamphetamine _meth.html.

Perrone J and Hoffman RS. (2000). Stimulants, cocaine, and amphetamines. In: *Emergency medicine: A comprehensive study guide.* Eds: Tintinalli JE, et al. McGraw-Hill, New York.; pp1113-1116

Winslow B, Voorhees K and Pehl K. (2007). Methamphetamine abuse. *American Family Physician; 76(8)*: pp1169-1174.

Chapter 8
Cocaine

"Cocaine isn't habit forming. I should know – I've been using it for years."

-Tallulah Bankhead

Cocaine is processed from the leaves of the *Erythroxylon coca* plant. The leaves are dissolved in hydrochloric acid to form cocaine hydrochloride. The cocaine can be mixed with ether, producing free base cocaine, or it can be extracted with sodium bicarbonate to form crack cocaine. The latter process is cheaper and easier to perform. Columbia is the number one producer of cocaine in the world. Cocaine was made illegal in the United States with the Food and Drug Act of 1906 and the Harrison Narcotic Act of 1914 (Hals & Richardson, 2001).

Neurobiology:

Cocaine can be insufflated nasally with the onset of action being 15 to 20 minutes, and the duration of action being 60 to 90 minutes. Cocaine may be smoked or injected with a peak in 5 to 10 minutes and duration of 30 minutes. These rapid highs are followed by intense crashes. Addicts will use in a binge fashion in order to avoid the crash. Cocaine binds to proteins to inhibit the re-uptake of dopamine, norepinephrine and serotonin. These elevated levels of neuro-amines create the sensation of euphoria. The euphoria is followed by a fall in the dopamine levels, resulting in depression and cravings. Cocaine stimulates the direct release of catecholamine from the adrenals, which stimulates sympathetic activity.

Metabolism:

Cocaine is **metabolized** in the liver and excreted by the kidneys. The active metabolites may be identified in the urine for 24 to 36 hours. Cocaine is frequently used with alcohol. The two substances combine to create **cocaethylene**, which has a longer half-life and increases the risk of sudden cardiac death (Hals & Richardson, 2001).

Effects:

Cocaine elicits a number of reactions; most are secondary to sympathetic activity (table 1.). Patients may be tachycardic, hypertensive, hyperthermia, tremulous and agitated. Cocaine may act as a type Ia sodium channel blocker and prolong the QT interval potentiating cardiac **dysrhythmias**. Beta-blockers are **contraindicated** in this situation. Beta-blockade will result in unopposed alpha stimulation and vasospasm, creating a hypertensive crisis. Benzodiazepines are the drugs of choice for cocaine induced tachy-dysrhythmias. Cocaine may cause **coronary ischemia** by coronary vasoconstriction, platelet aggregation, or by increased oxygen demand. The EKG may not be diagnostic, and cardiac enzyme analysis may be useful. The use of thrombolic therapy is controversial. Therapy is usually more conservative with the addition of benzodiazepines (Hals & Richardson, 2001). Beta-blockers and calcium-channel blockers are avoided.

Table 1. Signs of Cocaine Use
Dilated pupils
Tachycardia
Hypertension
Hyperthermia
Tremors
Agitation

Cocaine use carries a risk of **stroke**. Elevated levels of neuroamines cause vasoconstriction. Patients may present with hemorrhagic or ischemic strokes. 80% of hemorrhagic strokes have a pre-existing aneurysm or arteio-venous malformation. Cocaine abusers may present with **seizures**. They usually occur with in 90 minutes of last use. A cat scan should be obtained to rule out a stroke. Benzodiazepines should be used initially; phenobarbital may be used if there is no response (Hals & Richardson, 2001).

Table 2. Adverse Effects of Cocaine Use
Hypertensive crisis
Coronary ischemia
Dysrhythmias
Stroke
Seizures
Pulmonary compromise

Cocaine use is associated with several **pulmonary problems**. Cocaine use may result in reactive airway disease, pneumothorax, pneumomediastinum, and pulmonary edema. These problems are more common with crack use. There is also a disorder called **"crack lung"**. These patients present with fever dyspnea, hemoptysis, hypoxemia, chest pain, infiltrates and respiratory failure. This usually occurs 1 to 12 hours after use. Corticosteroids are the mainstay of therapy (Hals & Richardson, 2001).

"Cocaine washed-out" syndrome is commonly seen in the acute care setting. These patients present with a severe decrease in the level of consciousness and have no response to painful stimuli. The disorder is felt to be secondary to catecholamine depletion. Recovery is spontaneous and treatment is generally supportive (Hals & Richardson, 2001).

Cocaine use in **pregnancy** places both the mother and the fetus at risk. There is an increased chance of pre-eclampsia, eclampsia, placental abruption, premature labor and fetal death. Uterine rupture is not uncommon in mothers that have had a prior cesarean section. The fetus suffers from apnea and narcotizing enterocolitis (Hals & Richardson, 2001). Intrauterine cocaine exposure may also result in a decrease in the child's cognitive function (Singer, Arendt, Minnes, Farkas, Salvator, Kirchner & Kliegman, 2002).

Withdrawal:

Cocaine **withdrawal** does not pose a threat to the patient. The most dominant symptom is dysphoria. Desipramine has been used to treat the depression associated with the abstinent state. It is started at 50 mg daily, and titrated up by 50 mg every other day to a dose of 150 to 250 mg daily. This dose is maintained for a period of 3 to 6 months, and stopped with a 2 week taper (Miller & Gold, 1998). Propranolol may help the anxiety associated with cocaine withdrawal; increasing the likelihood that the patient will remain in treatment (Kampman, Volpicelli, Mulvaney, Alterman, Cornish, Gariti, Cnaan, Poole, Muller, Acosta, Luce & O'Brien, 2001). Amantadine may help to stabilize the disrupted dopamine system and diminish dysphoria (Kampman, Volpicelli, Alterman, Cornish & O'Brien, 2000).

References:

Hals G and Richardson W. (2001). Drugs of abuse and their complications: Emergency department evaluation and management: Part I. *Emergency Medicine Reports; 22(12)*: pp132-146.

Kampman KM, Volpicelli JR, Alterman AI, Cornish J, O'Brien CP. (2000). Amantadine in the treatment of cocaine-dependent patients with severe withdrawal symptoms. *American J Psychiatry; 157(12)*: pp2052-2054.

Kampman KM, Volpicelli JR, Mulvaney F, Alterman AI, Cornish J, Gariti P, Cnaan A, Poole S, Muller E, Acosta T, Luce D, O'Brien C. (2001). Effectiveness of propranolol for cocaine dependence treatment may depend on cocaine withdrawal symptom severity. *Drug and Alcohol Dependence 63(1):* pp69-78.

Miller NS and Gold MS. (1998). Management of withdrawal syndromes and relapse prevention in drug and alcohol dependence. *American Family Physician.; 58(1):* pp139-146.

Singer LT, Arendt R, Minnes S, Farkas K, Salvator A, Kirchner H and Kliegman R. (2002). Cognitive and motor outcomes of cocaine-exposed infants. *JAMA; 287(15):* pp1952-1960.

Chapter 9
Inhalant Abuse
"One man's poison is another man's drug."

-Ronald Knox

Certain volatile substances can be inhaled to create a "high" resulting in euphoria, loss of inhibition, relaxation and occasionally hallucinations. Inhalants are placed into three groups. Group I includes the volatile solvents, fuels, and anesthetics. This is the most commonly abused group. Group II includes nitrous oxide and group II includes the alkyl nitrites including amyl nitrate (Williams & Storck, 2007). These substances are commonly found in cleaning products, paints, adhesives and petroleum fuels. The vapors from these substances can be inhaled from the container ("**sniffing**"), poured on a rag and inhaled ("**huffing**") or poured into a bag and inhaled ("**bagging**"). "Bagging" is extremely dangerous, placing the user at high risk for asphyxiation (Hals & Richardson, 2001).

The Problem:

Inhalant abuse is a problem that is often missed in primary care. Inhalant abuse is popular with adolescents, as these chemicals are readily available, relatively inexpensive and legally obtained and have little "hangover" symptoms. The peak age of abuse is 14 to 15 years but the onset of use may be as early as 6 years (Williams & Storck, 2007).

Children with poor grades and low socioeconomic status are particularly vulnerable to becoming inhalant abuser (Williams & Storck, 2007).

Abusers will frequently look for products with warning labels, using these labels as a way to identify abusable substances. Poison control centers report approximately 8000 incidences per year with around 250 deaths per year. Nitrous oxide or "laughing gas" is usually diverted from medical and dental supplied and sold in gas filled balloons. It may be inhaled directly from aerosol cans containing whipped cream (Williams & Storck, 2007). Amyl nitrate "poppers" have become popular with the male homosexual community. The clinician needs to be alert for the signs of solvent use, including odors, stains on clothes, face and nails, sores on the mouth, recurrent epistaxis and behavioral changes (Table 1.) (White, 2000).

Table 1. Clues for Solvent Abuse
Odors
Stains on face and clothes
Sores on the mouth
Recurrent epistaxis
Behavioral changes

Effects:

The **organic solvents** are rapidly absorbed through the pulmonary vasculature and ultimately metabolized by the cytochrome P450 system. The chemicals retain their ability to function as solvents and will dissolve fats, including the myelin sheaths of neurons found in the central and peripheral nervous systems. These substances act as depressants having GABAergic effects while inhibiting glutamatergic neurotransmission (Williams & Storck, 2007). MRI studies have demonstrated consistent **abnormalities** of the thalamus, basal ganglion, pons and cerebellum in solvent abusers. These changes result in decreased short-term memory, delayed ability to learn and make associations, and extensive cognitive defects (Rosenberg, Grigsby, Dreisbach, Busenbark & Grigsby, 2002).

These addicts appear deviant even to individuals that suffer from other addictions. They lose the ability to control their behavior and they have complex denial systems, making treatment and recovery very challenging. These individuals may benefit from a comprehensive neurological rehabilitation program as well as substance abuse treatment. Nitrous oxide appears to act at the opiate receptors as well as having GABA mediated behavioral effects (Williams & Storck, 2007).

Nitrites differ in their mechanism of action. They have no direct central nervous system effects. They cause vasodilation and smooth muscle relaxation resulting in feeling lightheaded with enhanced sexual feelings, penile engorgement and anal sphincter relaxation (Williams & Storck, 2007).

The group I abuser will feel the effects of use with in minutes of inhalation and will demonstrate signs of **intoxication** for as long as five hours (Table 2.). They may present with slurred speech, diminished coordination, nausea, vomiting, headaches, reactive airway disease and decreased level of consciousness. They may also present with the social consequences of their drug use, such as poor school or job performance, and social maladjustment (Hals & Richardson, 2001).

Table 2. Signs of Solvent Intoxication
Slurred speech
Poor coordination
Nausea/vomiting
Bronchospasm
Decreased level of consciousness

Consequences:

Inhalant abusers are at risk for a number of medical consequences mostly associated with group I use (Table 3.).

Table 3. Consequences of Solvent Abuse
Encephalopathy
Dementia
Peripheral neuropathy
Dysrhythmias
Renal tubular acidosis
Reactive airway disease
Skin lesions
Fetal solvent syndrome

The solvents will cause white matter degeneration and atrophy, resulting in **encephalopathy** and **dementia**. They may present predominantly with cerebellar signs, such as ataxia, nystagmus and ocular flutter. Patients may also present with findings consistent with **peripheral neuropathy**. These substances will sensitize the myocardium to catecholamine creating a risk for lethal arrhythmia and **sudden inhalant death syndrome**. Individuals that abuse toluene can present with **renal tubular acidosis**. **Pulmonary manifestations** of inhalants are due to the irritant properties of the chemicals, resulting in laryngospasm and bronchospasm. **Dermatological** signs of use are secondary to the solvents dissolving the cellular membranes around the nose and mouth creating sores. Refrigerant abusers may present with frostbite around the nose and mouth. Solvent abuse while pregnant results in **fetal solvent syndrome**. These infants suffer from intrauterine growth retardation, cranial abnormalities, facial dysmorphia

87

and abnormalities of muscle tone. These infants may also have renal abnormalities (White, 2000). One issue often forgotten is the flammable nature of solvents. These substances can accidentally combust resulting in severe burns.

Chronic group II or nitrous oxide use may cause short-term memory loss and peripheral neuropathy. Nitrous oxide inactivates vitamin B_{12} resulting in **pernicious anemia-type syndrome**. Use of group II inhalants such as amyl nitrite can lead to hemolytic anemia if the abuser has glucose-6-phosphate dehydrogenase deficiency (Williams & Storck, 2007).

Treatment:

Treatment of **intoxication** is generally supportive. These patients should be given supplemental oxygen and placed on a cardiac monitor for 6 hours. Epinephrine is best avoided in these patients, as increased myocardial sensitivity to catecholamine may potentiate tachyarrhythmia. Patients in SVT or VT are best treated with a short acting beta-blocker such as esmolol (Hals & Richardson, 2001). Any other specific sequelae such as methemoglobinemia or burns should be addressed. The patient may need decontamination to avoid further intoxication and to prevent medical personnel from succumbing to the effects of fumes.

Chronic abusers of inhalants will suffer a non-specific, non-life threatening **withdrawal** syndrome. These patients tend to be irritable, jittery and diaphoretic, complaining of insomnia and nausea. They may be delusional and suffer from hallucinations. Treatment of withdrawal is typically supportive only (Anderson & Loomis, 2003). The treatment strategies for this type of addiction have not been fully elucidated. The standard principles of treatment are felt to be applicable with the addition of measures directed toward the associated neurocognitive defects and how these defects represent barriers to development of insight and bring unconscious motivations and actions to consciousness.

References:

Anderson CE and Loomis GA. (2003). Recognition and prevention of inhalant abuse. *American Family Physician 68(5)*: pp869-874.

Hals G and Richardson W. (2001). Drugs of abuse and their complications: Emergency department evaluation and management: Part II. *Emergency medicine reports; 22(13)*.

Rosenberg NL, Grigsby J, Dreisbach J, Busenbark D and Grigsby P (2002). Neuropsychologic impairment and MRI abnormalities associated with chronic solvent abuse. *J Toxicology 40(1)*: pp21-34.

White S. (2000). Abuse of inhalants. *Audio-digest Family Practice.48(18)*.

Williams, J. and Storck, M., and the Committee on Substance Abuse and Committee on Native American Child Health. (2007). Clinical Report: inhalant abuse. *Pediatrics; 119(5)*: pp1009-1017.

Chapter 10
Psychedelics and Selected Club Drugs
"Turn on, tune in, drop out"

-Timothy Leary

Neurochemistry of Psychedelics:

The use of psychedelic agents has been on the rise for the past several years. Agents with psychedelic properties are available in both natural and synthetic forms, sharing similar **pharmacological properties**. They act at the postsynaptic membrane of central serotonergic neurons to increase serotonin binding and enhance serotonin activity in the pontine raphe nucleus. This produces disinhibition in the occipital lobe and limbic system, resulting in illusions, visual hallucinations and bodily distortions. Dopamine is not affected, leaving reality testing intact (Giannini, 2000).

The Psychedelics:

Mescaline is a natural psychedelic that is found in the top of the peyote cactus. Mescaline has been used in Native American ceremonies for approximately 8000 years. It is not commonly abused because it readily causes nausea and vomiting, and has a very bitter taste. **Psilocybin** is a chemical produced by *Psilocybe* mushrooms found on cow manure. These mushrooms are generally found in the southeastern and northwestern United States. These mushrooms are frequently confused with more poisonous *Amanita* mushrooms resulting in severe toxic reactions. Psilocybin is heat stable allowing the abuser to cook the mushrooms while retaining their psychedelic properties. The Swiss chemist, Albert Hoffman, first synthesized lysergic acid diethylamide (LSD, acid) in 1938. The psychedelic properties of the substance were not discovered until 1943, when Dr. Hoffman spilled his discovery on his hands and had the first "acid trip" while bicycling home (Hals & Richardson, 1999).

Effects of Psychedelics:

These substances are ingested or, in the case of LSD, allowed to dissolve on the tongue. **Effects** are typically noted after 30 minutes and may last for 12 hours, with the peak activity occurring at around 4 hours post-ingestion (table). These patients will present with an increase in sympathetic tone, causing tachycardia, diaphoresis and pupillary dilation, as well as the classic distortions of reality. True psychotic episodes are rare but they do occur. Patients may suffer from "post-hallucination perceptual disorder" or "flashbacks" for months or years after drug use (Hals & Richardson, 1999). Treatment of intoxication is generally supportive. These patients do best in a quiet environment with minimal visual stimulation. Severely agitated individuals may benefit from treatment with a benzodiazepine. Ondansetron may alleviate agitation and psychosis by blocking serotonin receptors but this has not been proven. Chronic abusers do not undergo a true **withdrawal** syndrome with abstinence, but they may become dysphoric secondary to decreased serotonin activity. The dysphoria may be lessened with a selective serotonin re-uptake inhibitor such as Prozac (Giannini, 2000).

Table. Effects of Psychedelics
Tachycardia
Diaphoresis
Pupillary dilation
Distorted reality

Selected Club Drugs:

Club drugs have gained popularity with young people and with those attending "raves". They are believed to enhance social interactions by providing a sense of closeness, empathy and euphoria. These drugs include ecstasy which is akin to amphetamine and flunitrazepam, a benzodiazepine. These drugs are covered in their respective chapters. We will discuss ketamine, a dissociative anesthetic and γ-hydroxybutyric acid a sedative hypnotic.

Ketamine was derived from phencyclidine (PCP) in the 1960s. Ketamine is also known as "Special K, K, Kit Kat and Cat Valium". It inhibits neuronal uptake of norepinephrine, dopamine, serotonin and glutamate. The drug may be injected, inhaled or ingested. It has a rapid onset and the effects last 30 to 45 minutes. The user enters a dreamlike state with visual hallucinations and bizarre ideations. They often report out of body experiences and may have "flashbacks" days or weeks later. Physical effects include tachycardia, hypertension and hypopnea. Care is supportive focusing on the airway and respirations (Gahlinger, 2004).

γ-Hydroxybutyric acid (GHB) is called "G, Liquid Ecstasy, Soap, Easy Lay Cherry Meth and Georgia Home Boy" on the street. GHB is a natural product of GABA metabolism. It was first synthesized in 1960 as an attempt to create a GABA analog (Sneed & Gibson, 2005). It became popular as a nutritional supplement for bodybuilders in the early 1990s as a means of stimulating growth hormone release. In 2000 it was classified as a schedule I narcotic due to it being used as a "date rape" drug (Gahlinger, 2004). GHB inhibits GABAergic neurons via GABA$_B$ receptor mediation. It also inhibits presynaptic GABA release in the mesocorticolimbic dopaminergic system mediated by GHB receptors. This results in disinhibition of dopamine neurons and increased dopamine activity and reward resulting in addiction (Sneed & Gibson, 2005). The drug has a narrow margin of safety.

Overdose is manifested by rapid onset of coma, myoclonus, respiratory depression and bradycardia. Recovery is usually rapid and spontaneous. However, death may be the result of asphyxia, aspiration and pulmonary edema. Treatment is supportive focusing on the "ABCs" with airway protection and atropine as needed for bradycardia. There is no antidote and charcoal has no role in treatment (Sneed & Gibson, 2005). Overdose is more common in individuals concurrently taking protease inhibitors as both drugs utilize the cytochrome P-450 system for their metabolism. Alcohol ingestion also makes one vulnerable to overdose as both substances compete for alcohol dehydrogenase (Sneed & Gibson, 2005). Withdrawal for heavy GHB use is similar to the withdrawal of benzodiazepines and alcohol. Symptoms range from mild to full delirium and psychosis. Treatment is supportive and may require benzodiazepine taper (Sneed & Gibson, 2005).

References:

Gahlinger P. (2004). Club drugs: MDMA, γ-hydroxybutyrate, rohypnol and ketamine. *American Family Physician; 69(11)*: pp2619-2626.

Giannini JA. (2000). An approach to drug abuse, intoxication and withdrawal. *American Family Physician; 61(9)*: pp2763-2774.

Hals G and Richardson W. (1999). Drugs of abuse and their complications: Emergency department evaluation and management: Part II. *Emergency Medicine Reports; 22(13):* pp147-62.

Sneed O and Gibson M. (2005). Drug therapy γ-hydroxybutyric acid. *New England Journal of Medicine; 352(26)*: pp2721-2732.

Chapter 11
The Behavior of the Addict

"The mind in itself is its own place.
In itself, it can make a heaven of hell or a hell of heaven."

-Milton

The chapter on neurobiology described a number of neurochemical adaptations that occur with repeated exposures to substances of abuse. These neurochemical changes cause a predictable pattern of aberrant behaviors. A.A. calls this "a peculiar mental twist".

Freud's Topography:

Many of Sigmund Freud's theories including the Oedipal complex and penis envy have fallen out of favor. However, his theory of the topography of the mind appears to have a valid neurobiological basis. Behavior, thought and emotions stem from unconscious fears and desires as influenced by childhood experiences (Horgan, 1996). It appears that the dichotomy of psychology and neurobiology is false.

Freud's intrapsychic topography consists of the unconscious, preconscious and conscious thought processes. The unconscious is the repository of repressed thoughts directed by instinctual drives or primary process thinking. These processes involve the system of procedural or implicit memory located in the sensory cortices where stimuli are recognized and the amygdala, which is the site of acquisition of cued feeling states.

Implicit memories are concerned with habits such as drug use, perceptions and motor skills. (Kandel, 1999). Motives are hidden in the unconscious mind and may be withheld from consciousness by a repressive force (Solms, 2004).

The preconscious contains easily recallable memories. It is logical and based in reality (Solms, 2004). These memories are declarative or explicit in nature and reside in the medial temporal lobe and hippocampus (Kandel, 1999). The individual is not aware of most of the processes but has ready access to them as sensory percepts when attention is applied (Kandel, 1999). This action is mediated by the prefrontal cortex, which helps to bring explicit knowledge to conscious awareness by integrating sensory information with planned movement to create goal directed action. The conscious is directly connected to the external environment but has no direct connection to the unconscious (Solms, 2004).

The intrapsychic structures of psychoanalysis fall within this topography. Freud described the Id as the center of pleasure seeking and aggressive drives that uses unconscious primary process thinking with no direct influence from external reality. The Id appears to be the amygdala, which is the center of fear, rage, aggression, love, affection and mood. It wants what feels good. The Id also partially resides in the reticular formation and locus caeruleus of the brainstem that are responsible for emotional reaction such as the fight or flight response. The Superego resides in the dorsal frontal cortex consciously providing moral and legal guidelines. It is the personality's conscience wanting to do what is right. It should be noted that this region is adjacent to the ventral frontal cortex which controls selective inhibition and is felt to be the area responsible for the repression of motives from conscious thought (Solms, 2004). The Ego is the part of the mind that resides in the cortex and consists of unconscious rational processes that keep instinctual drives at bay to manage conscious experience. It is the referee between the Id and the Superego focusing on self-preservation and the appropriate application of the basic instinct (Solms, 2004).

Neurochemical adaptations and Freud:

Why bring up Freud? These areas are competing for control and in delicate balance. It doesn't take much for balance to be lost and the Id to gain power. This is what happens as a result of chronic exposure to substances of abuse. The use of drugs and alcohol stimulates the release of dopamine from neurons originating in the ventral tegmental area to post-synaptic neurons in the nucleus accumbens. This promotes CREB and δ-FosB activity strengthening neural pathways linking memories to the drug taking experience and increased reward. Chronic drug use results in depletion of dopamine and serotonin. The abstinent state results in elevated levels of CRF and norepinephrine creating distress, while the frontal lobe has little influence due to neurochemical changes. The addict is left with a physiologic imperative to use being enslaved by their primitive drives. They develop psychic conflicts due to this internal struggle. The Id or the devil on their shoulder is in control but the angel or Superego keeps talking filling them with guilt. Unconscious Ego defenses are employed to aid the psyche in this conflict by resolving, modifying or ignoring the conflicts helping to maintain a semblance of balance, safety and self. The defenses include denial, intellectualization, and repression to name a few. These defense mechanisms prevent information pertaining to the conflicts and drives from reaching the consciousness. Classical psychoanalysis calls this the dynamic or repressed unconscious (Kandel, 1999). The goal of psychotherapy is to aid the patient by helping them uncover and understand these defense mechanisms.

The Addict:

Craig Nakken's work, *The Addictive Personality*, describes the behavioral changes as a staged process of maladaptive behaviors (Nakken, 1996). In a sense this description explains how Dr. Jekyll transforms into Mr. Hyde.

Human beings have "**four natural relationships**". These relationships are formed between the individual and his family and friends, his self, his community, and his spiritual beliefs. Each of these relationships is structured around negotiation, and compromise. They form a support network that helps the individual in times of crisis. They also serve as a model for personal development and growth. Carl Jung calls this the "protective wall of the human community". The addict gets intimacy and intensity confused. They give up on the four natural relationships in favor of a more reliable source of pleasure, their drug of choice. Addiction is a pathological love relationship with a chemical or an action; anything that will quickly increase dopamine levels in their reward pathways. They try to meet their emotional and intimacy needs in an un-natural fashion. Their lives and actions revolve around manipulation of others and most importantly, themselves. This loss of connection results in spiritual bankruptcy, which becomes a tremendous source of pain and shame.

Stage I is the **internal change stage**. The addict begins to use the pleasurable sensation of the drug as an escape from life's problems. There is a negative conversion experience and the addict chooses the fantasy world created by the addiction over human experience. As dopamine and serotonin have not been depleted and corticotrophin releasing factor has not begun to elevate, the "pleasures" of substance usage out weight the pain. The addict is internally split regarding trust versus distrust of humanity. The dopamine rush begins to influence behavior, yielding acts of self-betrayal as cortical influences are over ridden by unconscious processes.

Character defects that begin to emerge in stage I:
Self-centeredness
False pride
Victimization
Dishonesty
Perfectionism
Resentfulness
Intolerance
Impatience
Envy
Wearing masks
Procrastination
Self-pity
Jealousy
Suspicious
Egotistical
Grandiosity
Greed
Lustful
Laziness

Self-respect and confidence decline. The addict loses the ability to connect with others and the addict begins to experience the painful consequences of these actions. The drug of choice worsens these feelings through **emotional amplification** secondary to monoamine depletion. An addictive ritual begins as "the self" starts to fight the addict. The addictive personality develops and Mr. Hyde emerges. The Id begins its battle with the Superego to gain supremacy yet the Ego remains relatively unscathed.

Stage II is the **life style change stage**. The addict's behaviors adapt to perpetuate the disease. These behaviors are termed "**survival skills**" by the recovery community. In reality these behaviors are distortions of thinking that allow the addict to rationalize their substance use and self-centeredness as the Id's shouts become louder.

15 Styles of Distorted Thinking/Defense Mechanisms
Filtering: You only see the negative in people and situations, and filter out the positive.
Polarized thinking: You see things as black and white. If you are not perfect you are a failure.
Over generalizing: You draw a conclusion with out all the facts. If something bad happens once, you expect it to happen repeatedly.
Mind reading: You assume to know how people are feeling and why they do what they do.
Catastrophizing: You expect the worst. You predict a negative out come.
Personalization: You take everything personally. You compare yourself to others, always trying to be one step better.
Control fallacies: Externally, you see yourself as a victim of fate and helpless. Internally, you feel responsible for the happiness and pain of everyone around you.
Fallacy of fairness: You feel resentful because you think you know what is fair but others won't agree with you.
Blaming: You either entirely blame yourself or others for every reversal of fortune. There is no shared accountability.
Shoulds: You have a list of rules that you and others must follow.
Emotional reasoning: You believe that what you feel

must be true.
Fallacy of change: You expect that other people will change if you pressure them enough. You need to change others because your happiness depends on them.
Global labeling: You generalize one or two qualities into a negative global judgment.
Being right: You believe that you are always on trial to prove that your opinions and actions are correct. Being wrong is unthinkable.
Heaven's reward fallacy: You expect to be rewarded for all of your sacrifice and are bitter when the reward does not come.

The addict becomes defensive regarding his/her substance use. The addict attempts to control others in order to reap personal benefit. This is when relationship problems develop. The addict is labeled by others and gives him/herself an attitude of victimization. There is a loss of behavioral control driven by neurochemistry. The pain of use now begins to outweigh the pleasure. Rituals begin to enslave the addict as he/she pulls away from the four natural relationships as the Id gains a foothold above the Superego and the addict becomes more conflicted with only the Ego defenses to maintain a limited connection with self.

Stage III is the **life breakdown stage**. The defenses lose their effectiveness. Intoxication loses its magic, as the pain greatly over rides the pleasure. As serotonin and dopamine depletion worsen, the patient becomes deeply depressed. The addict feels as if life is spinning out of control. Fears grow as coping skills breakdown. The addict lives in a state of anxiety, fear and rage. This corresponds to the elevation of corticotropin releasing factor in the amygdala. The addict interprets any stress-provoking situation as an abstinent state and uses substances to mask the pain. The addict is no longer able to identify with reality as the "self" has broken down and all defenses are depleted. The addiction is the only surviving relationship. Driven by instinct with diminished frontal lobe influence, they lose hope and become a suicide risk as the neurochemical changes affect cortical processing. They see the powerlessness in life and wish for an end to the pain. Dr. Jekyll murders Mr. Hyde.

The addict's behavior can be deviant even with abstinence from his/her drug of choice. These behaviors can be summed up into three general categories: being "bigger than the rules"; indicating grandiosity, and self-centeredness, "victimization" indicating self-pity, and resentments, "trying to fit a square peg into a round hole" indicating the attempt at control of other people and outside variables.

However, there is hope. The **recovery** process not only involves abstinence. The recovery process also involves re-modeling the individual's behavior to form a more functional pattern of living. These maladaptive behaviors are not only a source of chaos during the throws of addiction; they also represent a barrier to the recovery process. The addict's distorted perceptions, primarily **denial**, make education difficult. The addict may continue to see him/herself as a victim, and blame his/her problems on other people or circumstances. The addict may not be able to see these troubles as a consequence of substance use. When the addict faces the stresses of daily living he/she tends to be anxious and easily overwhelmed. These feelings may be misinterpreted as a withdrawal state and an elevation of CRF. They have learned through negative re-enforcement that substance use will decrease anxiety and their CRF levels fall. Therefore stress may be a trigger for relapse even after a period of abstinence.

Addicts tend to be individuals with a deep yearning for "the spirit". This may be why alcohol is referred to as spirits. They have a longing for **inter-connectedness**, but substance abuse has lead to isolation. The recovery process allows addicts to not only stop using mood-altering chemicals but to also under go behavioral change. This change allows addicts to rejoin society and to rebuild the four natural relationships. Addicts learn to drop their negative perceptual filters that were an obstacle to happiness and begin to see the world in a new positive light. They will learn the value of negotiation as opposed to the chaos created by manipulation. They learn to cherish the process of developing healthy relationships instead of harboring past resentments or predicting possible outcomes. Most importantly, the addict will choose to live in reality and discard the drug-induced fantasy in which they had been trapped.

References:

Horgan, J. (1996). Why Freud isn't dead. *Scientific American; 275(6)*: pp106-111.

Kandel, E. (1999). The biology and future of psychoanalysis: a new intellectual framework. *American Journal of Psychiatry; 156(4)*: pp505-524.

Nakken C. (1996). *The Addictive Personality: Understanding the Addictive Process and Compulsive Behavior*: 2d Ed: Hazelden Information and Education Services: Center City, Ma.

Solms, M. (2004). Freud returns. *Scientific American; 290(5)*: pp83-89.

Chapter 12
Childhood Scars

"Children begin by loving their parents.
After a time they judge them.
Rarely, if ever, do they forgive them."

-Oscar Wilde

There has been a great deal of debate regarding the origin of addiction. Is it nature or is it nurture? This question is much more complex than it appears on the surface. Methodological issues have plagued the scientific studies that have been undertaken by each camp. These issues include selection bias and failure to match control groups. However, there does appear to be strong evidence pointing toward a genetic or **hereditary basis** for a predisposition towards addiction. Adoption studies have shown that children of alcoholics brought up in a non-alcoholic home have an increased risk of alcoholism (Stabenau, 1985; Goodwin, 1982). Alcoholics have been found to have a genetic difference of the DRD2 receptor (Noble, 1993). This information is important, and it can help to relieve some of the guilt that may be tormenting the addict, but these are variables that cannot be changed.

The environmental side of the question is much more important when dealing with an individual that needs help. As addiction is a hereditary illness, the majority of individuals suffering from addiction grew up in homes with a parent that had an addiction (Searlesm, 1991). These families do not supply the nurturing structured environment that children need to grow into healthy adults. The child is left with a misperception of what is "normal" family life. These abnormal beliefs lead to chaotic relationships in adulthood and these beliefs need to be addressed if recovery is going to be obtained and maintained.

Early Childhood:

The relationship between the infant and the mother is the most important component of the early environment. The initial representation of people and relationships are critical for normal development. Age 0 to 2 or 3 years is the critical period that the infant must interact with a responsive environment for satisfactory development of the brain and personality. The attachment instinct organizes memory process and directs the infant to seek proximity to its mother. The parental response amplifies the infant's positive emotional states and soothes the infant's negative states. Repeated experiences are encoded into procedural memory to help the infant feel secure (Kandel, 1999).

The infant relies totally on unconscious procedural memory during the first two or three years as declarative memory has yet to develop. The infant will protest during brief periods of separation with anxiety and anger. This will last for minutes to hours and is associated with elevations of adrenocorticotropic hormone (ACTH) and glucocorticoids. Prolonged separation will result in sadness and depression with persisting hormonal elevations. Early adverse life experiences cause increased gene expression of CRF from the hypothalamus and the amygdala. This chronic high stress state will be imprinted in the procedural memory and impair declarative memory affecting the unconscious with subsequent neuroses (Kandel, 1999).

The Optimal Family:

The optimal family serves as a valuable source of **emotional support** and model of future behavior. It also serves as a model of how personal relationships should be cultivated. Members of the optimal family view the family as a system in which change is necessary and desirable. There are clear-cut boundaries between the family and the outside world as well as between individuals in the family. Major roles and functions are distributed within the immediate family, not the extended family. Parents share equally in power. Yet, children participate in decision-making and give feedback. Individuals within the family have a sense of identity and freedom of expression. This autonomy breeds accountability. Family members feel free to openly express emotions. Conflicts are resolved through empathic open communication. Tasks are dealt with by fair negotiation. The optimal family will grow and change as conditions demand.

The Dysfunctional Family:

The work of family therapist Virginia Satir illustrates that members of a family are all inter-connected, like it or not, in sickness and health. The personality theorist George Mead has written that our personal identity is equal to the sum total of our interpersonal relationships (Seitz, 1997). In essence, we are the products of our parenting. A child is not able to go through the natural stages of growth when raised in an addictive home. As an adult they are trapped in the fears and reactions of a child. These homes have **no consistency** in rules or discipline. The child is always "walking on eggshells". Not knowing if they will be met with praise or reprisals. They "learn" that they cannot do anything right and that something must be wrong with them. In an addicted household, the parent's actions cannot be questioned. The addicted parent "rules with an iron fist". The child learns that his/her wants and needs are secondary. Each child may begin to take on a specific role or roles that serve a specific purpose allowing the dysfunctional family unit to be held together (table).

Table. Roles in Dysfunctional Families
Dependent: This is the role of the addict. They are motivated by shame and use drugs or alcohol to relieve their pain. There is no benefit for the family.
Enabler: This is usually the significant other. They are motivated by anger and appear powerless. They take on the responsibilities of the family and become self-righteous.
Hero: This is typically the eldest child. They are driven by guilt and low self-esteem. They tend to be over-achievers. Their reward is positive attention and the family gains elevated worth. The price paid is a compulsive drive.
Scapegoat: This is usually a middle child that is driven by hurt. They tend to be delinquent and defiant. They get negative attention in return and they take the focus away from the dependent. These children are self-destructive and are at risk for addiction.
Lost child: This individual may also be a middle child. They are very lonely, isolated and shy. This helps them to escape their situation and allows the family to have one less member to worry about. This isolation tends to carry on to adulthood.
Mascot: This is usually the youngest child. They gain attention by being the family clown. They are hyperactive and serve the family as a source of entertainment. They grow into immature adults and tend to suffer from emotional illness.

To protect themselves they become people pleasers and seldom develop a personal identity as an adult (Adult Children of Alcoholics World Service Organization, n.d.).

Independence is viewed as a threat to the parent's authority. The parent will wield disparaging remarks to "put the child in his/her place". This decreases the child's self esteem even further, and the child learns not to excel to a level greater than the parent's level of success. The parent views this as a threat to their power. The child begins to subconsciously sabotage his/her own life and wonders why he/she continues to fail as this behavior continues into adulthood. The adult child continues to react in the way that allowed them to survive as a child. They will either defy authority, which can manifest in a **conduct disorder** or **antisocial behavior**, or suppress their own needs and attend to the needs of the person or people that represent their parents. If they choose the latter path, they feel guilty when they stand up for themselves. They may then begin to regard themselves as "door mats" (Adult Children of Alcoholics World Service Organization, n.d.).

As the child grows older, they begin to realize that their view of "normal" is a misconception. They tend to bond with individuals from dysfunctional backgrounds. This creates a cycle of **unhealthy relationships**, both romantic and non-romantic, that re-enforces their dysfunctional way of life. They were never taught about healthy boundaries. As a result, they are not able to set limits with themselves or others. They take on the opinions, needs and defects of others. They have no identities and must rely on being a "pathological chameleon". Early in the relationship, the adult child is not able to recognize this pattern. When the other individual's behavior becomes fully dysfunctional, the adult child feels betrayed. They may become depressed, self-loathing and take on the role of the **victim**. They may try to hold onto the relationship at all costs, terrified of emotional abandonment. Yet, they keep choosing partners that match their addicted parent. When they do get in a relationship that is relatively healthy, they tend to run and self-sabotage, feeling defective and undeserving (Adult Children of Alcoholics World Service Organization, n.d.).

The following is a list of behaviors compiled by the Adult Children of Alcoholics and Al-Anon (Al-Anon, 1984). These **behaviors** are typical for people that were raised in an addictive home.

Isolation, fear of people, and fear of authority figures.
Difficulty with identity issues related to seeking constantly the approval of others.
Frightened by angry people and personal criticism.
Have become an alcoholic, married one or both. A variation would be the attraction to another compulsive personality such as a workaholic. The similarity is that neither is emotionally available to deal with overwhelming and unhealthy dependency needs.
Perpetually being the victim and seeing the world from the perspective of a victim.
An overwhelming sense of responsibility. Concerned about the needs of others to the degree of neglecting their own wants and needs. This is a protective behavior for avoiding a good look at themselves and taking responsibility to identify and resolve their own personal difficulties.
Feelings of guilt associated with standing up for their rights. It

is easier to give into the demands of others.
An addiction to excitement. Feeling a need to be on the edge, and risk-taking behaviors.
A tendency to confuse feelings of love and pity. Attracted to people that they can rescue and take care of.
Avoidance of feelings related to traumatic childhood experiences. Unable to feel or express feelings because it is frightening and/or painful and overwhelming. Denial of feelings.
Low self-esteem. A tendency to judge themselves harshly and be perfectionistic and self-critical.
Strong dependency needs and terrified of abandonment. Will do almost anything to hold onto a relationship in order to avoid the fear and pain of abandonment.
Alcoholism is a family disease, which often results in a family member taking on the characteristics of the disease even if they are not addicted. Dysfunctional relationships, denial, fearful, avoidance of feelings, poor coping, and poor problem solving, afraid that others will find out what they are really like, etc.
Tendency to react to things that happen versus taking control and not being victim to the behavior of others or situations created by others.
A chameleon. A tendency to be, what others want them to be instead of being themselves. A lack of honesty with themselves and others.

In general, their survival motto is, "don't talk, don't trust, and don't feel".

These findings are not isolated to the addictive household. They may be found in homes with other reasons for dysfunction.

A parent may be suffering from some type of medical or mental illness that leads to a similar pattern of child rearing (Su, Hoffmann, Gerstein & Johnson, 1997). These types of histories need to be sought out when evaluating the addict seeking help, as this information can shed light on the origin of past dysfunctional behaviors.

Similarities to Borderline Personality Disorder:

It is interesting that these behaviors are very similar to those of borderline personality disorder. The following is the DSM-IV criteria for the diagnosis of BPD (American Psychiatric Association, 1994).

DSM-IV Criteria for Borderline Personality Disorder
Beginning by early adult life, the patient has unstable impulse control, interpersonal relationships, moods and self-image. These persistent or recurrent qualities are present in a variety of situations and shown by at least 5 of the following:
Frantic attempts to prevent abandonment, whether real or imagined
Unstable relationships that alternate between idealization and devaluation
Identity disturbance (severely distorted or unstable self-image or sense of self)
Potentially self-damaging impulsiveness in at least 2 areas such as binge eating, reckless driving, sex, spending, substance use (do not include suicidal or self-mutilating behaviors)
Self-mutilation or suicidal thoughts, threats or other behavior
Severe reactivity of mood creates marked instability (mood swings of intense anxiety, depression, irritability last a few hours to a few days)
Chronic feelings of boredom or emptiness
Anger that is out of control or inappropriate and intense (demonstrated by frequent temper displays, repeated physical fights or feeling constantly angry)
Brief paranoid ideas or severe dissociative symptoms related to stress

The **Dialectical Behavioral Theory** attempts to explain the behaviors of BPD as a result of childhood experiences. Studies have found a positive correlation between certain parental behaviors and BPD. These include a lack of consistency regarding punishment, and lack of validation of feelings (Linehan & Schmidt, 1995). Does this mean that ACoA behaviors and BPD are one in the same? It is possible and deserves further investigation.

Treatment:

Recovery from addiction is possible if an effort is made to treat these childlike patterns. These behaviors can continually resurface throughout the recovery process, sabotaging any progress towards a fulfilling life. Repeated failures in relationships, education and career can lead to feelings of hopelessness and despair. Life's challenges are repeatedly viewed through the negative perceptual filters created in childhood. The addict is not able to identify with his/her emotions, yet they act in an emotional childlike manner. There can be no growth when this is occurring. This is a setup for relapse. The first step in the recovery process is to help the addict chip through the denial and see these patterns of behavior to identify defense mechanisms and deal with internal conflicts. These issues are very complex and best handled by specialists in this type of therapy. The therapist will assist the addict in facing their oldest fears and to discover their own identity. There are a number of self-help groups (appendix 4) that can be a great service to the addict dealing with issues of growing up in an addictive home. They include Al-Anon and Adult Children of Alcoholics. These groups use a twelve-step model to help guide the individual in the process of self-discovery. They use the steps, meetings and the fellowship to share their experience, strength and hope with one another. They learn to release their parents of the responsibility for their actions today. They become their own parent and with the aid of their "higher power", their inner child is allowed to grow in a nurturing environment.

The healthcare provider must always keep in mind that these individuals are emotionally immature and may form unhealthy attachments to their caregivers. These therapeutic relationships commonly result in transference and/or counter-transference reactions, both of which will hinder progression in treatment. The provider must remain neutral in behavior and attitude and must keep his/her emotions modulated in times of crisis. Rules must be established, as these individuals have no concept of boundaries. Avoid excessive accommodation and favors. Establish a structured office environment. Provide definition, predictability and consistency with rigid adherence to interpersonal boundaries. Encourage structure in their lives as well. Be prepared for boundary violations from day one and acknowledge them in a neutral manner (Hubbard, Saathoff, Bernardo & Barnett, 1995).

The clinician must remember that the above dynamics not only occur in the addict's family of origin, but also occur in their current family. Therefore, the addict's family members should be referred for appropriate therapy.

References:

Adult Children of Alcoholics World Service Organization. (n.d.). *The Laundry List.* Accessed December 8, 2011 from: http://www.adultchildren.org/lit/Laundry_List.php

Al-Anon. (1984). *Al-Anon Faces Alcoholism.* New York, NY: Al-Anon Family Headquarters.

American Psychiatric Association. (1994). Diagnostic and Statistical Manual of Mental Disorders, 4th Edition. Washington, DC: American Psychiatric Association.

Goodwin DW. (1982). Alcoholism and heredity: Update on the implacable fate. In: Gomberg, et al., Eds., *Alcohol, Science and Society Revisited*, Ann Arbor, MI: University of Michigan Press. (pp. 162-170)

Hubbard JR, Saathoff GB, Bernardo MJ, Barnett BL. (1995). Recognizing borderline personality disorder in the family practice setting. *American Family Physician; 52(3)*: pp908-914.

Kandel, E. (1999). The biology and future of psychoanalysis: a new intellectual framework. *American Journal of Psychiatry; 156(4)*: pp505-524.

Linehan MM, Schmidt H. (1995). The dialectics of effective treatment of borderline personality disorder. *Theories in Behavioral Change.* Washington DC: American Psychological Association. (pp553-584)

Noble EP. (1993). The D2 dopamine receptor gene: A review of association studies in alcoholism. *Behavioral Genetics; 23(2)*: pp119-229.

Searles JS. (1991). Genetics of alcoholism: Impact on family and sociological models of addiction. *Family Dynamics of Addiction Quarterly; 1(1)*: pp8-21.

Seitz FC. (1997). Medical care and the family. In: Behavioral medicine made ridiculously simple. Miami: Med Master, Inc.

Stabenau JR. (1985) Basic research on heredity and alcohol: Implications for clinical application. *Social Biology; 32(3/4)*: pp297-321.

Su SS, Hoffmann JP, Gerstein DR, Johnson RA. (1997). Effects of home environment on adolescent substance use and depressive symptoms. *Journal of Drug Issues; 27(4)*: pp851-877.

Chapter 13
Uncovering the Specter of Addiction
"To know that one has a secret is to know half the secret itself."
-Henry Ward Beecher

The disease of addiction knows no boundaries. It crosses sexes, economic lines, social classes, educational levels and races. No one is immune to the disease of addiction. The addict does not typically look like a "skid row bum". The addict may look like the girl next door, your clergy, your child, your grandfather or your doctor. Because of this the clinician must maintain a high index of suspicion.

Clues:

Patients with addiction may present seeking recovery, but this is not very common. Their **denial** is usually too deep for them to see their substance abuse as a problem. These individuals will typically present with another complaint. There are a number of clues that point towards addiction as a source of the patient's difficulties (Figures1 & 2) (Schulz & Parran, 1998).

Figure 1. Complaints that may indicate substance abuse
Frequent absences from work or school
History of frequent trauma or injuries
Depression
Labile hypertension
Gastrointestinal symptoms
Sexual dysfunction
Sleep disorders

Figure 2. Findings suggestive of substance abuse
Tremor
Odor of alcohol
Tender hepatomegaly
Nasal irritation
Conjunctival irritation
Labile blood pressure
Tachycardia/arrhythmia
"After shave/mouthwash syndrome"
Odor of marijuana or solvents on clothing

Patients with full-blown addiction will demonstrate **behavioral changes**. They will classically be described as restless, irritable and discontent (see the chapter on behavior). Their attitudes will change as they begin to view the world through negative perceptual filters. Their performance at work or school may deteriorate. Their attendance may decline. Addicts also present

with complaints that are associated with the consequences of
their substance abuse (Figure 3.). The consequences of chemical
dependency usually follow a sequential pattern. Their job is
usually the last thing to go. They rely on employment as a source
of income to acquire their drug of choice.

Figure 3. Sequence of the Consequences of Addiction
1. Family & school
2. Social/isolation
3. Financial
4. Health
5. Legal
6. Job

Patients will present with **drug seeking** behaviors. These
patients attempt to pressure the physician to prescribe controlled
substances when the physician is hesitant to do so. These patients
tend to be manipulative and demanding. They may claim that the
only possible solution to their problem is a controlled substance,
and claim that non-addictive medications "don't work". They may
make statements regarding their high tolerance to medications.
Addicts often present with symptoms that do not correlate with
their physical findings. Drug seekers will come in stating that they
lost their prescription or their medications have been stolen. They
frequently try to pit one physician against another and attack a
resisting physician's pride. Some offer bribes or sex and others
threaten physical harm (Longo, Parran, Johnson & Kinsey, 2000).
The clinician must be alert to feelings associated with counter-
transference. These patients are certainly irritating but they are

driven by a physiological imperative to use. Their Id has gone wild as the Ego ignores the Ego-ideal presented by the Superego. All their Ego defenses stand ready to defend their disease. They view their drug of choice as the only "medication" that can help them to feel "normal". They are no more at fault than the individual that suffers from iron deficiency who is driven by pica to eat dirt.

Screening and Assessment:

The **Alcohol Use Disorders Identification Test** (AUDIT) is a ten-question screen used to identify the entire spectrum of problem drinkers and the **Short Michigan Alcohol Screening Test** (SMAST) is a screen for the consequences of alcohol use. These tests are primarily used in the research setting and are quite cumbersome (Foster, Blondell & Looney, 1997; Saitz, 2005). Screening for substance abuse is only as complicated as the clinician makes it. For drugs other than alcohol, simply ask, "What drugs do you use to help relieve stress?" Remember that there is no such thing as a social "crack" user or glue sniffer. The **"Quantity/Frequency Questionnaire"** is a good way to begin assessing a patient for alcohol abuse (Figure 4.) (U.S. Dept. of Health and Human Services, 1995).

Figure 4. The Quantity/Frequency Questionnaire
On average, how many days per week do you drink alcohol?
On a typical day when you drink, how many drinks do you have?
What is the maximum number of drinks you have had on a given occasion during the past month?

More than seven drinks per week or more than three drinks per occasion would indicate problem drinking for men and women over sixty-five years of age. More than fourteen drinks per week or more than four drinks per occasion indicate problem drinking for men and women under sixty-five years of age.

The next step in the evaluation would be to perform the **CAGE** or **TWEAK** questions. Both have proved to reliable tools for detecting alcohol dependence, though the TWEAK questions appear to be superior for evaluating women (Figures 5 & 6) (Ewing, 1984; Bradley, Boyd-Wickizer, Powell & Burman, 1998; Saitz, 2003). A limitation of these questionnaires is that they do not distinguish between past and current problems, but they have been found to be between 60 to 90 percent sensitive and 40 to 60 percent specific (Mersy, 2003).

Figure 5. CAGE Questions
Have you felt that you ought to **C**ut down on your drinking or drug use?
Have people **A**nnoyed you by criticizing your drinking or drug use?
Have you felt bad or **G**uilty about your drinking or drug use?
Have you ever had a drink or used drugs first thing in the morning (**E**ye opener) to steady your nerves, to get rid of a hangover or to get the day started?

Figure 6. TWEAK Questions
Tolerance: How many drinks can you hold? >=6 indicates tolerance and How many drinks does it take before you feel the effects? >=3 indicates tolerance
Worried: Have close friends or relatives worried or complained about your drinking or drugging in the past year?
Eye openers: Do you sometimes take a drink or a drug in the morning when you first get up?
Amnesia: Has a friend or family member ever told you about things you said or did while you were drinking that you could not remember?
Kut down: Do you sometimes feel the need to cut down on your drinking?
Scoring: 2 points each for tolerance or worried; 1 point each for eye opener, amnesia, or "kut" down

The next step is to review current life **stressors** and what the patient does to **cope** with the stressors. These stressors may include any of the consequences of substance use described above. The final step is to address any **family history** of substance abuse or other compulsive behaviors.

The **final assessment** is made when all this information is compiled. "At risk" drinking is indicated by, greater than fourteen drinks per week or greater than four drinks per occasion for men, and greater than eleven drinks per week or greater than three drinks per occasion for women. Or a CAGE or TWEAK score of one or higher for the past year, or a personal or family history of alcohol or drug problems. "Problem" drinkers have a CAGE or TWEAK score of one or two for the past year. Or alcohol/drug related medical problems. Or Alcohol/drug related family, legal or employment problems. "Dependency" is indicated by a CAGE or TWEAK score of three or four for the past year, or compulsion to drink. They exhibit loss of control over drinking/drugging, or relief drinking/using, or withdrawal symptoms, or increased tolerance (Samet, Rollnick & Barnes, 1996). Addiction is not dependent on counting drinks or snorts. Addition is a maladaptive pattern of behavior with continued use despite negative consequences.

Presenting the Diagnosis:

The patient should be told of the suspected diagnosis once the problem has been identified. This must be done carefully (Figures 7.) (Schulz & Parran, 1998). Any hope at progress towards recovery may be lost if the patient feels they are being labeled, judged or pressured. The clinician should state the suspected diagnosis and the facts supporting the diagnosis. Avoid any arguments and be prepared to bend with resistance. Have the patient return at a later date for further explanations if they are intoxicated.

Figure 7. Guidelines for Presenting the Diagnosis
Support: be empathetic and support the physician-patient relationship
Optimism: Patients expect to fail and need to hear a strong optimistic message
Absolution: The physician needs to re-enforce that their disease is not their fault
Plan: The treatment plan depends on the patient's readiness to change and needs to be a cooperative effort
Explanatory model: Get the patient's idea of their disease then try to explain it to them with an appropriate model.

References:

Bradley KA, Boyd-Wickizer J, Powell SH and Burman ML. (1998). Alcohol screening questionnaires in women. A critical review. *JAMA; 280*: pp166-171.

Ewing JA. (1984). Detecting alcoholism. The CAGE questionnaire. *JAMA; 252*: pp1905-1907.

Foster AI, Blondell RD and Looney SW. (1997). The practicality of the SMAST and AUDIT to screen for alcoholism amoung adolescents in an urban private family practice. *Journal of the Kentucky Medical Association; 95*: pp105-107.

Longo LP, Parran T, Johnson B and Kinsey W. (2000). Addiction: Part II identification and management of the drug- seeking patient. *American Family Physician; 61(8):* pp2401-2408.

Mercy, D. (2003). Recognition of alcohol and substance abuse. *American Family Physician; 67(7)*: pp1529-1532.

Saitz, R. (2005). Clinical practice; unhealthy alcohol use. *The New England Journal of Medicine; 352(6)*: pp596-607.

Samet JH, Rollnick S and Barnes H. (1996). Beyond CAGE: A brief clinical approach after detection of substance abuse. *Archives of Internal Medicine; 156(20)*: pp2287-2293.

Schulz JE and Parran T. (1998). Principles of identification and intervention. In: Principles of addiction medicine, 2nd Ed.: Chevy Chase, MD: American Society of Addiction Medicine, Inc.

U.S. Dept. of Health and Human Services, Public Health Service, National Institutes of Health, National Institute on Alcohol Abuse and Alcoholism. (1995). *The Physicians' Guide to Helping Patients with Alcohol Problems; publication no.*

95-3769. Bethesda, Md.: National Institutes of Health: NIH.

Chapter 14
The Dual Diagnosis
"An unexamined life is not worth living."

- Socrates

There is a strong association between addiction and other psychiatric disorders (Table 1.) (Liese & Chiauzzi, 1995). The mind doesn't exist without the brain and the effects of toxic exposure ravage the brain of the addict. The challenge lies in distinguishing the primary psychiatric diagnosis from the diagnosis that is secondary to the neurochemically-induced changes of substance abuse. Chronic use of the drugs of abuse can mimic nearly any psychiatric disorder.

Table 1. Increased risk of psychiatric disorders with drugs of abuse
Alcohol: 2.3 times
Marijuana: 3.8 times
Amphetamines: 6.2 times
Cocaine: 11.3 times
Opiates: 6.7 times
Barbiturates: 10.8 times

Acute intoxication and acute withdrawal of abused substances may also **mimic** a psychiatric disorder. Ideally, to make the diagnosis of a primary psychiatric disorder in the face of addiction the symptoms should persist after a period of three to four weeks of abstinence. It should also be noted that it might take up to a one year or longer for the neurochemical dysfunction to stabilize with chronic use of some substances.

There are a number of **clues** in the history that can aid in diagnosing a primary versus a secondary psychiatric disorder. Does the patient meet the full symptom pattern for the psychiatric diagnosis or are they suffering from isolated symptoms? What is the context of substance use? What is the temporal relationship of substance, symptom onset and critical life events? Is there a family history of psychiatric disorders? Is the history credible?

A psychiatric disorder will make recovery more difficult. These individuals tend to have disruptive tendencies, are more aggressive, and exhibit verbal hostility. They also lack coping skills and have difficulty managing practical responsibilities. These problems make it challenging for the individual to follow relapse prevention plans and to take simple suggestions. Appropriate referral and treatment can be undertaken if a potential psychiatric diagnosis can be identified.

Care must be taken when dealing with these individuals. If they sense any labeling or judgments, they will withdrawal and the interview will go nowhere. The clinician must sit quietly, listen attentively, be unhurried, and be sincerely empathetic. The diagnostic nature of the **interview** will deteriorate when the clinician interrupts prematurely to give reassurance and advice. If the individual gets acutely anxious, redirection to basic medical questions may be helpful. Questioning should be organized and goal oriented. It should begin with past medical and psychiatric histories. Life experiences are then addressed. These experiences include education, adoptions, relationships, divorces and deaths.

Then the family psychiatric history needs to be explored. The psychiatric screen may progress after the history has been obtained. The **"ABC's of the psychiatric patient"** is a useful tool for this purpose (Table 2.).

Table 2. The "ABC's of the psychiatric patient"
A: Anxiety disorders
B: Borderline and other personality disorders
C: Cognition
D: Depression and bipolar disorder
E: Eating disorders
F: Fighting
G: Gambling
H: Home violence
I: Indiscriminant sex
J: JOIMAT
K: Kill self

This information does not have to be gathered in one visit. In fact that could be overwhelming to the addict and the clinician. The following is a more in depth discussion of each category and the relationship to addiction and recovery. A positive response to any of the following screens may indicate the need for referral for more in depth psychiatric testing.

A: Anxiety Disorders

Anxiety disorders can be manifested as fear, agitation, palpitations and/or an impending sense of doom. Generalized anxiety disorder may simply be manifested as excessive or unwarranted worrying. These symptoms may be due to a primary disorder or they may be secondary to substance abuse. Acute exposure to stimulants such as cocaine and amphetamines will create a symptom complex that mimics anxiety. Acute withdrawal of depressants such as alcohol and benzodiazepines may present with the symptoms of anxiety. Individuals that have been chronically exposed to any of the substances of abuse will present with anxiety during a period of abstinence. This is due to an elevation of corticotropin releasing factor in the reward center of the brain that occurs in this setting.

The initial **screening** question should be, "Do you tend to be an anxious or nervous person?" Further questioning is needed to screen for specific anxiety disorders if the initial question has a positive response. For **generalized anxiety disorders** ask, "Do you tend to worry about things that you have no control over?" For **panic disorder** ask, "Do you ever experience a sudden rush of fear and nervousness that makes your heart pound and makes you afraid you're going to die or go crazy?" **Agoraphobia** needs to be ruled out if the patient gives a positive response to that question. Ask, "Have you had to limit where you go or what you do because of your anxiety?" A good question to screen for **obsessive-compulsive disorder** is, "Do you have rituals such as repetitive hand washing or repetitively checking to be sure your appliances are turned off before leaving your home?" To eliminate some of the false-positives, ask, "Do your compulsions interfere with your ability to live your life (Carlat, 1998)?"

If the patient is symptomatic after a period of abstinence or if they were symptomatic prior to the onset of their substance use a primary diagnosis should be considered and **treatment** instituted. Benzodiazepines should be avoided in those with addictions. BZDs act at the GABA receptors and will stimulate the reward pathway in addicts. This can greatly increase the risk of relapse. Buspirone is a good option for simple anxiety. For patients with associated insomnia, trazodone and imipramine may be beneficial. These agents have also shown an added benefit of slightly decreasing the chance of relapse. Selective serotonin re-uptake inhibitors are useful for patients with panic disorder and obsessive-compulsive disorder. Pindolol, a beta-blocker, can be used as an augmentation agent if panic symptoms persist despite SSRI therapy. The anticonvulsants valproic acid, gabapentin and carbamazepine have also been shown to be useful for patients with anxiety disorders (Gastfriend & Lillard, 1998). The atypical neuroleptics olanzapine, quetiapine and risperidone may be helpful for panic disorder and agoraphobia.

B: Borderline Personality Disorder and Other Personality Disorders

These patients present a challenge to the clinician. They have a high co-morbidity with other psychiatric disorders and high rates of suicidal ideation. They tend to violate boundaries and behave in a hostile manner if they do not get their way. This is a common problem in addicts that have grown up in addictive homes (see the chapter "Childhood Scars"). The mnemonic "**I DESPAIRR**" (Figure 1.) is a useful way to remember the criteria for BPD (Carlat, 1998).

Figure 1. The Diagnostic Criteria for Borderline Personality Disorder
Identity problem
Disordered affect
Empty feeling
Suicidal behavior
Paranoia or dissociative symptoms
Abandonment terror
Impulsivity
Rage
Relationship instability

Most of this information will become evident by obtaining a **relationship history**.

Rigid boundaries must be maintained with these patients. As a fear of abandonment is a core symptom they may demand an excessive amount of time and support. These individuals may benefit from cognitive-behavioral therapy or dialectical-behavioral therapy (Dimeff, Comtois & Linehan, 1998). Patients may also benefit from Al-Anon if they grew up in an addictive home. Any co-morbid diagnosis must also be addressed.

The other personality disorders may be present in the addicted individual. It will be helpful to identify these patients, as their symptoms can be a barrier to communication as well as recovery. "**BAD SHAPE**" is a useful mnemonic for recalling the various personality disorders (Figure 2.) (Good & Nelson, 1992).

Figure 2. The Personality Disorders and Core Symptoms
Borderline: see above
Antisocial: habitually break the law
Dependent: rely on others for guidance and emotional support
Schizoid: aloof, withdrawn, difficult to engage
Schizotypical: have odd and nearly psychotic behaviors
Histrionic: exaggerate and respond with strong emotions to relatively minor difficulties
Avoidant: show attachment to others but shy away from social relationships
Paranoid: suspicious of others but not psychotic
Passive aggressive: use passivity to express anger
Empathic (Narcissistic): can't empathize, usually extremely vain, can't admit being wrong

C: Cognition

Abuse of substances such as MDMA and inhalants may result in cortical dysfunction and cognitive defects. The post-acute withdrawal syndrome of alcoholism and alcoholic dementia may also cause cognitive problems. Substance abuse in the elderly is also a problem in today's society. These patients may have an underlying primary diagnosis of dementia. These patients should be screened for memory impairments and cognitive status. The **"JOIMAT"** mental status exam is a useful screen for this setting, though formal cognitive testing is indicated for positive results due to a relatively high rate of false positives. This tool will be discussed later in this chapter. Organic and metabolic etiologies need to be explored as well. Patients with cognitive dysfunctions may require specialized psychological referral for cognitive behavioral therapies. Patients with a primary diagnosis of dementia may benefit from treatments such as tacrine and donepezil if they are in the early stages of the disease.

D: Depression and Bipolar Disorder

Mood disorders may be secondary to acute use of depressants such as alcohol, barbiturates, and benzodiazepines. The symptoms may also be from acute withdrawal of stimulants like cocaine and amphetamines. Chronic exposure to the substances of abuse may also cause depression due to neuroamine depletion. The diagnosis of mood disorder may also be a primary diagnosis, though this is a difficult diagnosis to make. **Cognitive theory** states that these individuals hold on to the fantasy that bad things should not happen to them. They hold on to their childhood narcissism. They selectively perceive the negative aspects of life and believe that they should be exempt. A good screening question is: "Have you been depressed?" If the response is positive, the next step is to identify any associated neurovegetative symptoms. These can be remembered by the mnemonic "**SIGECAPS**" (Figure 3.) (Carlat, 1998).

Figure 3. The Neurovegetative Symptoms of Depression
Sleep disorder: increased or decreased
Interest deficit: anhedonia
Guilt: worthlessness, hopelessness, regret
Energy deficit
Concentration deficit
Appetite disorder: increased or decreased
Psychomotor retardation or agitation
Suicidality

The diagnostic criteria for **major depression** are a depressed mood or anhedonia with four of the neurovegetative symptoms for at least two weeks. The diagnostic criteria for **dysthymic disorder** are two of the neurovegetative symptoms and depression for at least two years.

It is important to screen for **bipolar disorder** as symptoms of this disorder greatly increase the chances of relapse. The initial screening question should be: "Have you had periods of feeling so happy or energetic that your friends told you that you were talking too fast or that you were too hyper?" The other cardinal symptoms of bipolar disorder need to be explored if they give a positive answer. The presence of elevated or irritable mood plus three of the seven cardinal symptoms make the diagnosis of mania. "**DIGFAST**" (Figure 4.) is a useful mnemonic in this case (Carlat, 1998).

Figure 4. The Cardinal Symptoms of a Manic Episode
Distractibility: inability to focus
Indiscretion: excessive involvement in pleasurable activities such as sex and spending
Grandiosity
Flight of ideas
Activity increase
Sleep deficit: decreased need for sleep
Talkativeness: pressured speech

The **treatment** of mood disorders in the addicted population does not vary that much from the non-addicted population. Higher doses of the selective serotonin re-uptake inhibitors may be needed in alcoholics. This is because of the activation of the microsomal enzyme activating system that occurs with chronic alcohol exposure. Desipramine is a good choice for individuals addicted to cocaine, as it has been shown to decrease the relapse rate. This appears to be because it increases the sensitivity of the dopamine receptors. The medication dose needs to be started low and increased slowly as it can be activating. Valproic acid and carbamazepine are good choices for the treatment of bipolar disorder. Care must be taken to monitor the patient's hepatic enzymes, especially with alcoholics and patients with hepatitis (Brady, Myrick & Sonne, 1998).Depressed patients may benefit from making a **gratitude list**. They are asked to list all of the things about themselves and their lives that they consider good. This forces them to look past the negative and see the positive aspects of life.

E: Eating disorders

The co-morbid nature of eating disorders and substance abuse was first noted in the 1970's. 12 to 18% of people with **anorexia nervosa** are also substance abusers. 30 to 70% of people with **bulimia nervosa** abuse substances. Food and the drugs of abuse appear to fulfill the same reinforcement and motivational function in the mesocorticolimbic reward system. **Compulsive overeaters** have been shown to have a decreased number of DRD2 receptors, the same defect noted in people with addiction. The density of DRD2 receptors negatively correlates with the body mass index. Identification of the compulsive overeater can usually be accomplished with simple observation of their weight and obtaining a dietary history. Identification of the other disorders is not as straight forward. The "**SCOFF**" questionnaire is a useful screening tool (Figure 5.) (Morgan, Reid & Lacey, 1999).

Figure 5. SCOFF Questions
Do you make yourself Sick because you feel uncomfortably full?
Do you worry you have lost Control over how much you eat?
Have you recently lost more than One stone (14 pounds) in a three-month period?
Do you believe yourself to be Fat when others say you are too thin?
Would you say that Food dominates your life?

Two or more positive responses are a likely indication for anorexia or bulimia, and further investigation is warranted.

The **treatment** of eating disorders requires a multidisciplinary approach. They need intensive behavioral treatment as well as nutritional education. These patients commonly have medical complications that also need to be addressed. Exercise has been shown to increase DRD2 receptor density and may benefit the compulsive overeater (Vastag, 2001). Exercise should be used with caution for the other disorders, as excessive exercise may be one of their symptoms. Selective serotonin re-uptake inhibitors may be of benefit to bulimics. No pharmacological treatments have been shown to be beneficial for anorexics.

F: Fighting

Repeatedly getting into fights may be a **warning sign** for a number of disorders especially in the adolescent population. These disorders include, conduct disorder, **intermittent explosive disorder**, and anti-social personality disorder in the post adolescent. The full symptom complex should be explored and the behaviors need to take place at times when the patient is not under the influence. "**FAR PUT**" is a useful screen to help uncover a diagnosis of conduct disorder (Figure 6.).

Figure 6. "FAR PUT": Findings Consistent with Conduct Disorder
Fights: Circumstances and how many?
Active sexually: Age of first sexual experience?
Running away from home: Overnight? How many times?
Police: Harming people or animals, vandalism, theft?
Use of substances: Alcohol, tobacco, or drugs? Frequency & duration of use?
Truancy, suspensions or expulsions

Individuals that carry these behaviors beyond adolescence are diagnosed with anti-social personality disorder. People that grow up in homes with parental substance abuse, psychiatric illness, marital conflict, abuse and neglect are at particular risk. The common feature is inconsistent parental availability and discipline. These individuals see no consistent relationship between their behavior and the consequences of their behavior

Some patients will have the isolated symptom of sudden aggressive outbursts without provocation. They do not pre-contemplate their violent acts. They just "snap". The diagnosis of **intermittent explosive disorder** must be considered for these individuals. These patients do not show a pattern of rule breaking or illegal behavior.

Co-morbid substance abuse must be addressed first. A **positive reward system** needs to be established for appropriate behavior and there must be clear consequences for inappropriate behavior. These patients need a structured daily routine and may benefit from structured recreational activities. The parents of adolescents with conduct disorder with need counseling for parental techniques and proper communication. There are several pharmacological treatments that may help the impulsive nature of these individuals. Bupropion and the SSRI's have been shown to decrease their aggressive-impulsive behaviors. The anticonvulsants, carbamazepine and valproic acid, can decrease aggressiveness. Clonidine decreases impulsivity and aggression, but it may cause depression and sedation (Searight, Rottnek & Abby, 2001).

G: Gambling

Pathologic gambling appears to have a high co-morbidity with addiction. 10% of heavy drinkers have been shown to suffer from pathologic gambling and 18 % of alcoholics have at least one gambling related problem. Pathologic gamblers also have a high rate of personality disorders. The etiology of pathologic gambling is unclear, but they have been shown to have a defect in the DRD2 gene similar to people with addiction. This implies that they also have a defect in the **mesocorticolimbic-dopamine system** that may prevent them from experiencing natural pleasure. Gambling may serve as a way to elevate the dopamine levels in the reward pathways, resulting in a "high". The tolerance and withdrawal symptoms exhibited by pathologic gamblers substantiate this. The person with addiction is destined for relapse if he/she continues to gamble and seek this artificial pleasure.

The "**LIE/BET**" questionnaire is an easy tool to screen for gambling related problems. It consists of two simple questions: "Have you ever had to **lie** to people important to you about how much you gambled?" and "Have you ever felt the need to **bet** more money?" A more detailed gambling history should be obtained if the individual gives a positive answer to one of these questions. "**OWE BIG DEBT**" is a useful mnemonic to remember the diagnostic criteria of pathologic gambling (Figure 7.). Five or more positive responses would indicate the diagnosis.

Figure 7. Diagnostic Criteria for Pathologic Gambling
Overly occupied with thoughts of gambling
Weaseling money from others to gamble
Escape emotions by gambling
Bogus efforts at controlling or stopping gambling
Irritable or restless when not gambling
Gambles to chase losses
Debt concealment by lying
Embezzlement, fraud, forgery, or theft
Botched career, education, marriage, or relationships secondary to gambling
Tolerance: needs to gamble increasing amounts to achieve desired "high"

Gamblers Anonymous is a twelve-step program of recovery modeled after Alcoholics Anonymous. It is a spiritual program that, with the aid of a higher power, helps the patient to overcome their irrational thoughts and to "restore them to sanity". Behavioral, cognitive, and cognitive-behavioral therapies are quite important for these patients. The goal is to challenge and correct the patient's irrational thoughts and to identify the reasons for gambling and to confront any defenses and loss chasing behaviors (Unwin, Davis & DeLeeuw, 2000).

H: Home violence

Substance abuse is a known risk factor for domestic violence. This seems to represent an association of one common social problem with another problem. There appears to be no direct cause and effect connection. **Domestic violence** is a pathological wheeling of power within a household. The abuse can be manifested in a number of ways including; physical abuse, emotional abuse, sexual abuse, economic abuse, intimidation, threats, and isolation. These behaviors may be perpetuated against the partner or against any children in the home. Domestic violence crosses all racial, socioeconomic, religious and ethnic groups. Although partner violence most commonly is male toward female, it may also be female toward male and it can occur in homosexual couples. A history of prior or current abuse must be explored. Victims of any type of abuse may be rout with shame, guilt and resentment. These emotions are a potential trigger for relapse and need to be addressed as early as possible in recovery (Eyler & Cohen, 1999).

The most dangerous form of abuse is physical abuse or battering. Lenore Walker has identified the three phases of the **battering cycle**. The first phase is the tension build up phase.

There is an escalation of psychological abuse and interpersonal tension during this period of time. The second phase is the explosion or acute battering phase. This phase marks the period of acute violence and the resulting physical trauma. The inciting event does not need to be of any great importance. A simple spark can ignite a large explosion. The final phase is the resolution or contrition phase. The batterer attempts to show remorse, but it is usually not genuine as their narcissism prevents them from seeing any wrongdoing. This is done in an effort to prevent the family from breaking apart. The victim will usually accept the apology and remain in the home. The victim may begin to "pick fights" earlier in the cycle to prevent the escalation of the batterer's emotions (Seitz, 1997).

Sexual abuse, even if remote, leads to a life of turmoil from the emotional scars. Sexual abuse includes any act of incest, molestation, assault or rape. The abuse may or may not include overt violence. Short-term behavioral symptoms include; mood disorders, sleep disorders, genital pain, sexually acting out, truancy, and running away. Long-term consequences include: delinquency, substance abuse, poor relationships, prostitution, promiscuity, guilt, shame, depression, post-traumatic stress disorder, and social withdrawal.

The victims of sexual abuse may undergo any of a number of adjustment patterns. These patterns are a form of psychic self-preservation. **Avoidance** is when the patient refuses to acknowledge or discuss the event. They experience self-blame, guilt and self-doubt. If the individual is a child he/she may be fearful of adults. **Repetition** is revisiting the victimization by sexually acting out, continued self-blame, frequent anxiety, and poor relationships with peers and family. These individuals may experience conversion reactions. They will demonstrate emotional distress in a more socially acceptable physical symptom. The victim may identify with the perpetrator in order to cope with the trauma. These people will become antisocial and angry. They may also exhibit sexually deviant behavior, maintain relations with the perpetrator, and blame authorities. **Integration** is the healthiest of the adjustment patterns. The victim effectively copes with the trauma and the resulting emotions. He/she will blame the perpetrator and not blame his/herself (Seitz, 1997b).

It is very important to screen for past and current abuse. Failing to do so can increase the feelings of isolation and discourage any efforts to seek safety. The "**SAFE**" questions are a useful tool for identifying abuse and focus on safety and empowerment of the victim (Figure 8.) (Neufeld, 1996).

Figure 8. The SAFE Questions
Stress/Safety What stress do you experience in your relationships? Do you feel safe in your relationships/marriage? Should I be concerned for your safety? Did you ever feel unsafe or threatened as a child?
Afraid/Abused Are there situations in your relationships where you have felt afraid? Has your partner ever threatened or abused you or your children? Have you been physically hurt or threatened by your partner? Has your partner forced you to have sexual intercourse that you did not want? Where you ever threatened or abused as a child?
Friends/Family If you have been hurt, are your friends or family aware of it? Do you think you could tell them if it did happen? Would they be able to give you support?
Emergency plan Do you have a safe place to go and the resources you and your children need in an emergency situation? If you are in danger now, would you like help in locating shelter? Would you like to talk with a social worker, a counselor or me to develop an emergency plan?

Expect the patient to be torn between sharing with you and being "loyal" to their partner. Be empathic but remember to distance your feelings and values. Relate the abuse pattern to the victim as a form of **cognitive therapy**. Do not hesitate to make referrals to the appropriate community, legal, and counseling services. Community based trauma groups are a valuable resource for empowerment. They can guide the patient along the path from victim to survivor.

It is also important to identify the **abusers** when they are seeking help for chemical dependency. Abusive behavior is the result of multiple factors, including individual characteristics, a family history of violence, and a cultural background that condones violence as a means for dealing with problems and as a means to control women. These patients will have to deal with a tremendous amount of shame and guilt after the drug induced "fog" clears and they can see past their narcissism. The shame may be too much if these issues are not dealt with and growth is not obtained. Referral to specialized psychotherapy is indicated. **Funneling** is a technique that is used to progressively expose a history of violence. This method begins with less threatening questions and progresses to more direct, specific questions (Figure 9.) (Eyler & Cohen, 1999).

(Figure 9.) The Funneling Technique
"Tell me about your relationship with your partner?"
"People have different ways of showing disagreement or anger in relationships. Sometimes people talk loudly, shout, threaten, hit or use weapons. How do you show anger and disagreement to your partner?"   Wait for a response, then ask:
"Anything else?" or "And then what happens?"   Repeat until patient offers nothing else.
Probe for specific types of violence: "Have you ever yelled at your partner?"   "Have you ever demeaned or berated your partner?"   "Have you ever destroyed your partner's property or other things?"   "Have you ever forced unwanted physical or sexual contact on your partner?"   "Have you ever pushed or hit your partner?"   "Have you ever threatened your partner with a weapon?"   "Have you ever hurt your partner with a weapon or object?"

Abuse, even if it was in the remote past, leaves deep, unyielding emotional scars.

One of the more devastating sequelae is **post traumatic stress disorder** or PTSD. PTSD arises following exposure to perceived life-threatening trauma (abuse, assault, rape, MVA, combat). The patient may become symptomatic immediately after the trauma and the symptoms may resolve after several months, or they may become symptomatic after more than six months and the symptoms may last indefinitely. One third of individuals with PTSD may remain symptomatic after ten years. If the patient relates a history of trauma then a more detailed symptomatic history should be obtained. "**DREAMS**" is a useful mnemonic for remembering the symptoms of PTSD (Figure 10.) (Lange, Lange & Cabaltica, 2000).

Figure 10. Symptoms of PTSD
Detachment: Detached from the event or relationships. Numbing of emotional responses.
Re-experiencing the event: In the form of nightmares, recollections or flashbacks.
Event had emotional effects: Threatened life or loss of physical integrity. Feelings of helplessness or disabling fear.
Avoidance: Of places, activities or people that are a reminder of the event.
Month in duration: Symptoms last more than one month
Sympathetic hyperactivity or hypervigilance: Insomnia, irritability and poor concentration.

Benzodiazepines have classically been the **treatment** for PTSD. They should be avoided for patients with addictions, as there is a great potential for abuse and triggering relapse. The SSRI's have been shown to reduce all three clusters of PTSD symptoms; re-experiencing, avoidance and hypervigilance. These agents may also help with any co-morbid diagnosis. Trazodone has SSRI properties and serotonin blockade effects. It will help with any associated insomnia and help to augment the action of the SSRI. Trazodone also suppresses rapid eye movement sleep and which will help to reduce nightmares. Anti-adrenergic agents are useful for alleviating sympathetic hyper-activity. Clonidine, propanolol and guanfacine can reduce nightmares, hypervigilance, startle reactions and rage (Lange, Lange & Cabaltica, 2000). The atypical neuroleptics may also benefit these patients. Cognitive-behavioral therapy, group therapy and systematic desensitization are important adjuncts for these patients.

I: Indiscriminant Sex

The relationship history may uncover a history of indiscriminant, deviant or compulsive sexual behavior. This may be an indication of a sex or love addiction. 83% of sex addicts have concurrent addictions. Therefore; it is very likely that you will see these patients as they seek treatment for their chemical dependency. **Sexual addiction** is a persistent and escalating pattern of compulsive sexual behavior (Figure 11.) that is acted out despite increasing negative consequences to self and others (Figure 12.). These behaviors interfere with normal living and cause severe stress on family, friends, loved ones, and work.

Figure 11. Addictive Sex Behaviors
Compulsive masturbation
Multiple affairs
Consistent use of pornography
Unsafe sex
Sexual anorexia
Multiple or anonymous partners
Phone, cybersex
Sexual massage, escorts, prostitutes
Prostitution

Figure 12. Consequences of Sex Addiction
Social
Relationship
Emotional
Legal
Physical
Financial

There is a very high correlation between **childhood abuse** and sex addiction. In one study, 72% had been physically abused, 81% had been sexually abused, and 97% had been emotionally abused in childhood. These factors may indicate a potential etiology for the disorder.

The **sexual addiction cycle** describes what happens in the psyche of a sex addict (Figure 13.). A pain agent starts the cycle.

The emotional distress causes a separation between the self and the feelings. This is called disassociation. As the disassociation becomes more severe they enter an altered state. They lose touch with reality and sexually acting out makes sense. They have no insight to potential consequences, they act on their compulsion. This is the pursuing behavior stage. They may make a phone call or try to find a prostitute. This ultimately leads to the behavior in question. The sexual act leads to an elevation of endorphins, which cause an increase of **dopamine** in the pleasure center of the brain, creating a very short-lived "high" that numbs the emotional pain. These patients experience a great deal of shame secondary to their behaviors. The shame acts as a pain agent and perpetuates the cycle. **Sexaholics Anonymous** describes the feeling as follows; "This produced guilt, self-hatred, remorse, emptiness and pain, and we were driven ever inward, away from reality, away from love lost inside ourselves (Sexaholics Anonymous, 2001)." These patients will experience **tolerance** and **withdrawal**, which will increase the frequency and intensity of their sexual acts. Their behaviors change and they pull away from the four natural relationships like people with chemical addictions.

Figure 13. The Sexual Addiction Cycle
A Pain Agent: Begins the cycle of addiction, Emotional Discomfort, Unresolved Conflict Stress, A Need to Connect
Disassociation: Separation between yourself and your feelings
Altered State: Reality gets blocked out
Pursuing Behavior: Moving towards acting out
Behavior: Acting out
Time: Period before cycle begins again
Disassociation: Separation between yourself and your feelings

Love addicts are "hooked" on the thrill of new relationships (Figure 14.). They confuse romance, intensity and sex with love. They move from one "romance" to another as each becomes "safe" and loses its excitement. They are consumed with seeking out new relationships, thinking that this will be the one that cures all their pain. Their relationships are full of dependency, guilt and abuse. They leave a path of destruction and negative consequences (Weiss, 1998).

Figure 14. Signs of Love Addiction
Constantly seeking out a sexual partner, new romance or significant other
An inability or difficulty in being alone
Consistently choosing partners who are abusive or emotionally unavailable
Using sex, seduction and intrigue to "hook" or hold onto a partner
Using sex or romantic intensity to tolerate difficult experiences or emotions
Missing out on important family, career or social experiences in order to maintain a romantic relationship
When in a relationship, being detached or unhappy, when out of a relationship, feeling desperate and alone
Avoiding sex or relationships for long periods of time to "solve the problem"
An inability to leave unhealthy relationships despite repeated promises to self or others
Returning to previously unmanageable or painful relationships despite promises to self or others
Mistaking sexual experiences and romantic intensity for love

The "**Sex/Relationship CAGE**" is a simple screen when a sex or love addiction is suspected. "Have you felt the need to **C**ut back on your sexual activity/relationships?" "Do you get **A**ngry if someone comments on your sexual activity/relationships?" "Have you felt **G**uilty secondary to your sexual activity/relationships?" "Do you use sex/relationship to cope with **E**motions?"

The **treatment** of sex and love addictions is similar to the treatment of chemical addictions. Treatment is best performed with the assistance of a specialized counselor with the aid of a twelve-step group such as Sexaholics Anonymous. The treatment begins with a "**detox**" period. The patient will experience a **withdrawal** syndrome consisting of irritability and poor concentration. The patient will be able to use this time to examine their prior behaviors and motivations, once the withdrawal has ended. A written contract of appropriate sexual/relationship behavior is useful. The next step is "de-traumatizing". Several things are addressed during this phase. Past abuse issues need to be identified and dealt with. Pain agents also need to be identified. The patient needs to be able to recognize pain agents and learn to effectively cope with these stressors to avoid the activation of the addictive cycle. The patient will need to regain the ability to relate to their feelings and recognize disassociation at its onset. This is also the time when the patient is taught how to rebuild the four natural relationships. The final phase is centering. This is when the sex addict learns to "live life on life's terms". They can stop the cycle if they can deal with their emotions and their pain in the first or second stages of the addictive cycle (Weiss, 1998b; Bissette, 1995).

J: JOIMAT

"**JOIMAT**" is a useful way to remember the mental status exam. This exam can uncover cognitive defects (as discussed earlier) and psychosis. The subject of this section will be psychosis. **Psychosis** is the loss of touch with reality. Psychosis may be a primary or secondary diagnosis. The temporal relationship with substance use and the onset of symptoms is helpful. If the patient is hallucinating, the type of hallucination is also helpful (Figure 15.) (Good & Nelson, 1992).

Figure 15. Types of Hallucinations
Olfactory: Temporal lobe seizures or most other causes
Auditory: Schizophrenia or bipolar disorder
Visual: Organic brain syndrome
Tactile: Stimulant abuse or alcohol withdrawal

Screening questions for psychosis are best blended in with other portions of the interview. For example: "Depression sometimes causes people to have strange experiences, like hearing voices or feeling that others are trying to harm them. Has that happened to you?" "When you misplace things, do you sometimes think that they've been stolen?" "Have you ever heard or seen people coming into your house?" "Have drugs ever caused your mind to play tricks on you, like seeing things or having paranoid ideas?" "Have people been harassing you or trying to harm you?" Psychosis should be suspected if a positive response is given to any of these questions. A more detailed mental status exam will help to tease out a possible diagnosis (Carlat, 1998).

Judgment is the ability to understand acceptable patterns of behavior and the consequences of unacceptable patterns of behavior. To assess judgment, ask; "If you found a stamped envelope in a gutter, what <u>should</u> you do with it?" To place it in a mailbox is the correct response.

Orientation is the awareness of person, place and time. Time disorientation is commonly seen with organic brain syndrome. Patients with severe organic brain syndrome may be disoriented to person. Disorientation to place is less common with organic brain syndrome.

Intellectual function is the assessment of the patient's cognitive state. The patient's education must be taken into account, and questioning should take this into account. This portion of the evaluation will also assess attention span and concentration. The level of function may be decreased with organic brain syndrome and depression. Have the patient subtract serial sevens from one hundred. Have them subtract serial threes from fifty if they have less than a high school education. Ask the names of the current and past four presidents.

Memory should be assessed at three levels. Long-term memory can be evaluated by asking the patient to recall distant life events such as their marriage. Short-term memory is assessed by having the patient recall three unrelated objects after a five-minute period. Immediate recall may be evaluated by asking the patient to repeat six digits forward and backward.

Appearance may give you many clues to possible psychiatric problems. What is the patient's affect? How is the patient dressed? Does the patient appear disheveled? Is the patient extremely neat? Does the patient have any visible scars or tattoos? Is there a tremor or other signs of agitation? What is the patient's speech like?

Examination of **thought** content and processes may yield useful information. Thought can be assessed by having the patient interpret a proverb such as; "People that live in glass houses should not throw stones." This can uncover logical vs. concrete vs. bizarre vs. loose associations. This line of questioning may also uncover paranoia.

Psychosis is a tremendous barrier to recovery and is a significant challenge for the clinician. Appropriate psychiatric referral should be made with the suspicion of psychosis. The atypical neuroleptic agents are commonly used for these patients. Cocaine addicts may benefit from the addition of an augmentation agent such as desipramine, mazindol or amantadine (Ziedonis & Wyatt, 1998). These agents help to elevate dopamine levels in the brain and can aid in treatment. The group Dual Recovery Anonymous can help these patients once they have been symptomatically stabilized. This group uses a twelve step spiritual program to address concurrent psychiatric and substance abuse issues.

K: Kill Self

Patients with addictions and psychiatric disorders will commonly contemplate **suicide**. They may come to a point in their lives that there seems to be no end to their pain. The chaos and turmoil they experience becomes more than they can bear. They see suicide as the only way to end their pain (Figure 16.) (Seitz, 1997c). They choose a permanent solution to a temporary problem.

Figure 16. Suicide Risk Factors
Sex: Females more attempts, males more successful
Age: greater than forty
Depression: See no end to the pain
Previous attempts:
Ethanol and drug abuse: Loss of reasonable thought
Resent loss of an important relationship: Feel alone in the world, painful
Social support lacking:
Organized plan for self destruction: Lethality
No spouse: Single persons at greater risk
Sickness: Debilitating illness, feel like a burden

Asking patients about suicidal ideation does not encourage them to commit suicide. All patients with addictions should be **screened** with a simple question. "Sometimes when people feel sad or depressed or have problems in their lives they think about suicide. Have you ever thought about suicide?" Further questioning is indicated if the patient gives a positive response (Figure 17.) (Gliatto & Rai, 1999).

Figure 17. Questions for Suicidal Ideation
"How long have you had suicidal thoughts?"
"Did anything in your life trigger these thoughts?"
"What keeps you from killing yourself?"
"Do you have a plan for killing yourself?"
"Do you own a gun?"
"Do you have access to dangerous medications?"
"Have you 'practiced' your suicide?"
"Have you changed your life insurance policy or will?"
"Have you given away any of your possessions?"

These added questions might give an indication of the lethality of the suicidal thoughts. The patient should be hospitalized if they have a plan and a means to commit suicide. The patient may be able to avoid hospitalization if they do not have a means and if they will contract for safety. These patients and patients that do not have a plan should be evaluated for psychiatric disorders and stressors.

References:

Bissette D. (1995). The nature of sex addiction. Accessed December 9, 2001 from: http://healthymind.com/s-theory.html.

Brady K, Myrick H and Sonne S. (1998). Co-morbid addiction and affective disorders. In: *Principles of addiction medicine, 2nd Ed.* Chevy Chase, Md.: American Society of Addiction Medicine, Inc.

Carlat AJ. (1998). The psychiatric review of symptoms: A screening tool for family physicians. *American Family Physician; 58(7)*: pp1617-1624.

Dimeff LA, Comtois KA and Linehan MM. (1998). Borderline personality disorders. In: *Principles of addiction medicine, 2nd Ed.* Chevy Chase, Md.: American Good WV and Nelson JE. (1992). Psychiatry Made Ridiculously Simple. Miami: Med. Master, Inc.

Eyler AE and Cohen M. (1999). Case studies in partner violence. *American Family Physician;* 60(9): pp2569-2576.

Gastfriend DR and Lillard P. (1998). Anxiety disorders. In: *Principles of addiction medicine, 2nd Ed.* Chevy Chase, Md: American Society of Addiction Medicine, Inc.

Gliatto MF and Rai AK. (1999). Evaluation and treatment of patients with suicidal ideation. *American Family Physician; 59(6)*: pp1500-1506.

Good WV and Nelson JE. (1992). Psychosis. In: *Psychiatry made ridiculously simple.* Miami: Med. Master, Inc.

Lange JT, Lange CL and Cabaltica RBG. (2000). Primary care treatment of post-traumatic stress disorder. *American Family Physician; 62(5):* pp1035-1040.

Liese, B.S., and Chiauzzi, E. (1995). Alcohol and drug abuse. *Home Study Self-Assessment Program.* American Academy of Family Physicians (AAFP) Monograph 189. Kansas City: AAFP.

Morgan JF, Reid F and Lacey J. (1999). The SCOFF questionnaire: assessment of a new screening tool for eating disorders. *BMJ; 319*: pp1467-1468.

Neufeld B. (1996). SAFE questions: overcoming barriers to the detection of domestic violence. *American Family Physician; 57(8):* pp2575-2580.

Searight HR, Rottnek F and Abby SL. (2001). Conduct disorder: diagnosis and treatment in Primary care. *American Family Physician; 63(8)*: pp1579-1589.

Seitz FC. (1997). Domestic violence, in: *Behavioral medicine made ridiculously simple.* Miami: Med Master, Inc.

Seitz FC. (1997b). Sexual abuse, in: *Behavioral medicine made ridiculously simple.* Miami: Med Master, Inc.

Seitz FC. (1997c). Suicide: "Oh God, is there no one to listen?" In: *Behavioral medicine made ridiculously simple.* Miami: Med Master, Inc.

Sexaholics Anonymous (2001). *The Problem.* Accessed December 9, 2001 from: www.sa.org/problem.php.

Unwin BK Davis MK and De Leeuw JB. (2000). Pathologic gambling. *American Family Physician; 61(3)*: pp741-748.

Vastag B. (2001). What's the connection? No easy answers for people with eating disorders and drug abuse. *JAMA; 285(8)*: pp1006-1007.

Weiss R. (1998). *Love Addiction Part One - The Problem.* Accessed December 9, 2001 from: http://love-addiction.com/add1.html.

Weiss R. (1998b). *Love Addiction Part Two - Recovery.* Accessed December 9, 2001 from: http://love-addiction.com/add2.html.

Ziedonis D and Wyatt S. (1998). Psychotic disorders. In: *Principles of addiction medicine, 2nd Ed.* Chevy Chase, MD: American Society of Addiction Medicine, Inc.

Chapter 15
The Stages of Change and Motivational Interviewing
"When the eyes say one thing and the tongue another,
a practiced man relies on the language of the first."
- Ralph Waldo Emerson

The goal of **recovery** is not mere abstinence from drug use. Recovery is a drastic change in lifestyle and behavior. Addicts will **mourn** over their old way of life and will go through the grieving process: denial, anger, bargaining, depression and acceptance. Addicts, by nature, have a tremendous fear of change and will resist the prospect of change. They do not respond well if they feel they are being backed into a corner. Effective communication is the key to retaining these patients in treatment and motivating them to pursue a healthier and happier lifestyle.

Communication:

Communication typically occurs at three levels and a clinician caring for addicts needs to be aware of all three. The **cognitive level** of communication is that which encompasses logical thinking with the focus on content. This would include questions, which should remain open-ended, sensitive and tactful. Paraphrasing or restatement may be used to clarify any confusion regarding the point the patient is trying to make. Short phrases, such as "I see", may be used to encourage the patient to continue. Silence is also a form of intellectual communication. Silence may be a time for self-examination, obtaining new insights or avoiding an issue.

The **emotional level** of communication can help to gain access to not only the events in a patient's life, but also to the patient's reactions to the events. "Emotional paraphrasing" is a tool used to diminish the intensity of the patient's feelings, while communicating warmth and understanding. Colorful speech and analogies that are consistent with the patient's culture and vocabulary may help to capture the emotional tone of a conversation.

The **transactional level** of communication is very important when dealing with addicts. The **Transactional Analysis Model** theorizes that each individual's psyche is made up of an "adult", a "child" and a "parent". Any number of transactions is possible when two people communicate. There will be little problem when people communicate at the same level. Trouble is inevitable with cross-transactions. Addicts will become extremely defensive if their doctor takes the role of a parent and lectures them for their behavior or substance use. The ideal transaction occurs at the adult to adult level (Seitz, 1997).

Dr. Carl Rogers has identified four factors that help to establish effective therapeutic relationships. First, the clinician must consider all channels of communication including speech, facial expressions and body language. The clinician must be genuine, personable and friendly. The clinician does not have to agree with the patient's point of view, but the clinician should try to accept their point of view. Most importantly, the clinician should be empathic (Seitz, 1997). **Empathy** is not an emotional state of feeling sympathy or compassion. Empathy is a type of understanding. It is listening to the total communication, verbal, non-verbal and emotional, and letting the patient know that they are being understood. This sense of understanding is comforting and helps to relieve isolation. It is rare for addicts to get this type of understanding and this, alone, may be all that is needed to gain trust and open their minds to new ideas. The professional must be careful not to cross the line to sympathy. Sympathy may be interpreted as patronization and cause them to withdrawal from the interaction (Platt & Platt, 1998).

Stages of Change:

Change does not happen overnight. It is not an isolated event. Change is a staged process that occurs overtime. When trying to aid in motivating change in an individual, it is necessary to identify which stage of change the patient resides. Interventions can then be made that are appropriate to that patient's stage. The **pre-contemplation stage** is when the patient is not even thinking about change. They may believe that the consequences of usage are not serious. The addict may be in denial ("Don't Even No I Am Lying") regarding drugs or alcohol being the origin of their problems. They may be resigned to the feeling that they will fail any attempted change. They may feel that they have no control over their actions.

Addicts begin to see that their difficulties could be due to substance use when they reach the **contemplation stage**. This is when patients will start to weigh the pros and cons of their behavior and the suggested change. This is a time of ambivalence. Their ambivalence is normal, not pathological.

Addicts are in the **preparation stage** once they realize the benefits of making the change and begin to explore how to make the change. Individuals at this stage may experiment with small changes, such as drinking only beer or changing their drug of choice.

With the right direction, the patient will then move to the **action stage.** This is when the person is ready to seriously consider or take definitive action towards making change.

The **maintenance stage** begins once the addict has made a genuine effort to recover. Addiction is a disease that is noted for its relapses and it is very seldom that the initial effort to change is permanent. Any relapses need to be dealt with in a positive light to avoid discouragement. These people tend to be self-deprecating and any negativity may cause them to pull back and sink further into their addiction. Relapses need to be taken as an experience that will aid in learning and growth. "Those that do not learn from the past are doomed to repeat it (Zimmerman, Olsen & Bosworth, 2000)."

Motivation:

Motivation is not a personality trait or a defense mechanism. Motivation is a probability factor that the patient will do what is needed to pursue a healthier lifestyle. Motivational interviewing is a technique that is employed to assist patients to recognize and address their present or potential problems. It is intended to help resolve ambivalence and direct them on the path of change. When done properly the addict presents the arguments for changing. Change arises from within rather than being imposed from external pressure. It is important for the clinician to understand the stages of change and use this information as a guide to approach the addict. Learning the principles behind motivational interviewing is much more important than learning scripted questions and phrases. Addicts may pick up on the scripting and interpret that as the clinician not being genuine. The FRAMES model is a general way of approaching patients that need to make a change in their lives (Figure) (Graham, 1998).

The FRAMES Model
Feedback: Give personalized feedback appropriate to the patient's stage of change. Discuss drinking patterns and attempt to correlate with consequences.
Responsibility: Emphasize that it is the patient's responsibility to change. This must be done in a non-judgmental fashion. This will give the patient a sense of empowerment. They are not responsible for their disease, but they are responsible for their recovery.
Advice: Provide clear advice to reduce and/or stop drinking, but remember the choice is up to the patient and they will most likely resist. Move on in an empathic, non-judgmental fashion if resistance is met. The addict will give indications when they are in the contemplation and action stages.
Menu: Brainstorm with the patient to create a menu of options of how to affect the desired change.
Empathic: See above. Remember empathy does not

equal agreement or approval.
Self-efficacy: Support the patient. Addicts lead a life that has resulted in repeated failure. It is easy for them to become discouraged and self-loathing. These people need praise when they succeed and encouragement when they have setbacks. Remind the patient that the goal is "progress, not perfection".

Progressing Toward Change:

The **Readiness to Change Ruler** is a useful tool for assessing the patient's readiness to change and what barriers to change exist. It consists of a simple straight line drawn on a sheet of paper that represents a continuum from "not prepared to change" on the left to "ready to change" on the right. The patient is asked to place a mark on the line that corresponds to their current position in the process of change. The clinician can then ask why they did not place the mark farther to the left. This will give you a sense of the patient's current motivation. Then ask want would it take to move the mark farther to the right. This will give clues to perceived barriers to change. The clinician can then brainstorm with the addict to identify potential ways to overcome these barriers (Zimmerman, Olsen & Bosworth, 2000)."

It is important to open with non-threatening dialogue when the addict is in the **pre-contemplation stage**. Asking about their lifestyle rather than asking about their alcohol or drug usage can do this. Ask them; "What's going on in your life?" or "Tell me what your typical day is like." The individual may be able to see for their self that there is a problem with their behavior. This is also a good time to ask the addict; "What does your drug use do for you?" and "What would you like from life?" A discrepancy between their present behavior and their broader goals may become evident to them. Clarifying their goals and allowing the patient to explore the potential consequences of their behavior can amplify the discrepancy. However, it is imperative that the clinician does not take the role of the parent. It is easy to lecture these patients. Lecturing only evokes resistance and arguments, and may even escalate substance usage. The professional must keep in mind that the goal is for the patient to realize that change is needed (Kushner, Levinson, Miller & Maher, 1998). Ambivalence may be overcome with a simple experiment. Suggest that the patient take one drink a day, no more, no less, for one-month. Let them know that it is practically impossible for an alcoholic/addict to do this because of their neurochemistry. Their lack of success may direct them towards change.

The clinician can help the addict move from the **preparation** to **action stage.** Use the Readiness to Change Ruler to identify what is keeping the patient from making the desired change, then brainstorm for possible solutions. The patient is invited to consider new information and is offered new perspectives. The professional must be prepared to "roll with resistance". Addicts are "master manipulators" and will do anything to avoid what they fear (False Evidence

Appearing as Reality) (Kushner, Levinson, Miller & Maher, 1998).

It is just as important to be involved when the patient is in the **maintenance stage** as it is in the earlier stages. Addiction is a disease of remissions and relapses. Have the patient identify what happened if they relapse, then work with them to identify methods that will help to avoid further relapses. This may be a good time to encourage twelve-step involvement. If the addict is involved in a twelve-step program, advise them to meet with their sponsor to review their program prior to the relapse and what triggered the relapse (Kushner, Levinson, Miller & Maher, 1998).

Addicts are a difficult population to work with. They have many behavioral traits that create fear and resistance to change. The clinician must remember that the addict's ambivalence is not pathological and they are not threatening the professional's expertise. Interactions will go much smoother if they remain at the adult-to-adult level, if the clinician is empathetic and if the clinician does not apply judgments or labels.

References:

Graham A. (1998). *Motivational interviewing*. From a lecture: Case Western Reserve University School of Medicine; February 1998.

Kushner PR, Levinson W, Miller WR and Maher L. (1998). Motivational interviewing: What, when, and why. *Patient care; 32(14)*: pp55-72.

Platt FW and Platt CM. (1998). Empathy: A miracle or nothing at all. *Journal of Clinical Outcomes Management; 5(2)*: pp30-33.

Seitz, FC. (1997). Doctor patient communication. In: *Behavioral medicine made ridiculously simple*. Miami: Med Master, Inc.

Zimmerman GL, Olsen CG and Bosworth MF. (2000). A "stages of change" approach to helping patients change behavior. *American Family Physician; 61(5)*: pp1409-1416.

Chapter 16
Stress and Addiction: Useful Behavioral Tools
"Those things that hurt, instruct."

- Benjamin Franklin

People instinctively react to stress in one of two ways. They will fight manifested by anger or aggression or they will take flight marked by fear and escape. Fight or flight depends on what has worked and what has not worked in the past. Genetic vulnerability and neurochemical reserve also play a role. Addiction, by its very nature, breeds an enormous amount of stress. This may be a consequence of substance use or dysfunctional behavior. Unmanaged stress is a risk factor for relapse. Stress comes from both internal and external sources. **External** sources of stress include physical illness, work issues, school issues, financial pressures or family difficulties. More subtle external sources include the weather, noise, traffic or overcrowding. **Internal** sources of stress are created by how the addict psychologically responds to the external stressors (Newburg & Newburg, 1998).

Vaillant's hypothesis states that poor adaptation to stress, not the stress itself, is what causes ill health (Stuart & Lieberman, 1993). The neurochemical and subsequent behavioral changes associated with addiction leaves the patient with very poor coping skills. Addicts are conflicted with complex defensive mechanisms, tending to be self-centered and self-seeking, with unrealistic expectations of life. Pride, guilt and fear drive their reactions. They attempt to control situations and others, rather than "accepting the things they cannot change".

This yields a self-perpetuating cycle, resulting in more stress and chaos. The patient's perceptual filters and social support systems are the mediators of the stress response (Seitz, 1997). **Perception** is the meaning assigned to a stressor. Addicts look at life as if "the glass was half empty". Negative perceptual filters paint a bleak picture and result in hopelessness, fear and other negative emotions. These emotions are typically based on past experience, not the current situation, and may cloud perceptions. Addicts have burned most of their bridges by their aberrant behaviors. Social support is essential to minimize the negative impact of stress. Strong support systems are a venue for venting and a resource for positive feedback.

Physiology:

The **physiologic response** to stress closely resembles the response to priming and withdrawal of various abused substances. The stress response is mediated by the hypothalamic-pituitary-adrenal axis, which activates the sympathetic nervous system resulting in the release of epinephrine, norepinephrine and cortisol mobilizing energy and increasing cardiac tone (Sapolsky, 2003). This causes tachycardia, elevated blood pressure, tachypnea, dilated pupils, and inhibition of digestion, increased perspiration and impaired immune function. Brief exposure to stress will increase dopamine levels in nucleus accumbens.

Repeated or chronic exposure to stress hormones without a buffer leaves the individual in a state of being on guard and hypervigilant (Sapolsky, 2003). Dopamine levels will rapidly decline. The locus caeruleus will become depleted of norepinephrine causing psychomotor retardation. Then serotonin levels drop adversely affecting mood and the ability to sleep (Sapolsky, 2003). Chronically stressed people will eventually experience fatigue, lightheadedness, headaches, insomnia, anxiety, or depression while stressed. Stress will affect memory, concentration, thought processes and creativity (Newburg & Newburg, 1998). Practicing addicts in an abstinent state have elevated levels of corticotropin-releasing factor (CRF) within the amygdala, the center of fear as well as pleasure. CRF has anxiogenic properties. The preconscious allows sensory information to bypass the cerebral cortex and affect the amygdala prior to conscious awareness. Any sensory input that has be unconsciously linked drug use and relief of distress will trigger a craving (Sapolsky, 2003). This is a reflection of implicit or procedural memory giving the Id strength. Addicts are conditioned by negative re-enforcement to use when they feel these symptoms. They give in to the Id and take flight or a chemical escape from the stress rather than fighting the Id and remaining abstinent. Therefore, it is important to recognize stress as a tremendous threat to sobriety.

Evaluation and Management:

The clinician can provide a huge service to these individuals by helping them to identify stressors and develop healthy coping strategies. The professional can serve as a source of social support and offer suggestions to modify the patient's perceptions. "**DENUP**" is a tool that is useful for evaluating stress (Figure 1.).

Figure 1. Clinical Assessment of Stress: "DENUP"
Demands: Task demands, emotional demands, life events
Expectations: Excessive expectations of self, of others, of control
Needs: Need for power, achievements, affiliations, affection, finances
Uncertainty: Controllable, uncontrollable, and uncertain
Perspective: Values, meaning, purpose (i.e. spiritual base)

Have the patient make a list for each category. Have them include methods that they would use for coping with each stressor. The patient should return to review the list and coping techniques. The clinician can use this as an opportunity to brainstorm with the patient and develop alternative coping strategies as needed. This is also a good opportunity to assess the patient's perceptions and offer insight to distortions in thinking. Do one category a week to avoid overwhelming the addict (Frank, 1993). Discuss ways to pursue actions and choices that can prevent repeating patterns that create stress. There are many techniques that can be suggested for stress management (Figure 2.) (Newburg & Newburg, 1998; Seitz, 1997). Twelve-step programs are a valuable resource for the stressed out addict. These programs are a place to gain insight and social support.

Figure 2. Stress Management Techniques
Progressive relaxation: decrease muscle tension, decrease sympathetic tone
Exercise: increase serotonin levels, increase DRD2 receptors, improve self image
Proper nutrition: avoid hyper/hypoglycemia, maximize internal resources
Guided imagery/creative visualization: improve positive perceptions
Hypnosis: improve positive perceptions
Biofeedback: decrease sympathetic tone
Recreation: distraction
Prayer and Meditation: decrease muscle tension, decrease sympathetic tone, gain insight, spiritual enhancement
Yoga: decrease muscle tension, improve flexibility, and decrease sympathetic tone, spiritual enhancement
Tai Chi: decrease muscle tension, improve flexibility, and decrease sympathetic tone
Message therapy: decrease muscle tension
Plenty of sleep: maximize internal resources
"The Stress Management Workbook": gain insight
Local stress management programs and workshops: gain insight

Prevention of stress may be the greatest lesson that addicts can learn in early sobriety. Have the patient **H.A.L.T.** to avoid stress accumulation. Addicts should not allow themselves to become too hungry. **H**unger can precipitate hypoglycemia, which may be interpreted as an abstinent state and result in cravings. The addict needs a balanced diet to provide them with the nutritional resources needed to cope with daily challenges. Anger can act like a cancer eating away at the addict. Anger causes individuals to focus on themselves and their pride may trigger them to act out on their old addicted models of behavior. This may lead to remorse or guilt, feeding their negativism, leading relapse. Loneliness and isolation are two of the primary findings in addiction. This creates boredom and cuts the addict off from the recovery community. If addicts allow themselves to become too tired they will not have the required energy to cope. They will be easily overwhelmed.

Brief Therapy:

Emotional problems are prevalent in addicts and there will be times when individuals will come to you in **crisis**. They will be so stressed that their coping resources will become overwhelmed, creating a psychological and spiritual dilemma. These patients will become less effective, less efficient and unable to solve problems. This is a time of danger and a time of opportunity, as they become open to intervention. Society has granted professionals several "**social powers**" (Figure 3.).

Figure 3. The "Social powers" of Physicians
Reward Power: The professional has health resources needed by the patient
Coercive Power: Power to make people feel uncomfortable
Expert Power: Knowledge of medicine and behavior
Referent Power: Act as a role model or an example
Legitimate Power: Contracted doctor-patient relationship

Because of these "powers", clinicians are able to use words to influence the psyches of patients to help them gain insight or change behaviors. This is called **psychotherapy**. The goal of psychotherapy is to aid the patient return to a level of functioning consistent with, or even above, societal norms (Newburg & Newburg, 1998). There are several elements essential for successful psychotherapy. There must be an established therapeutic alliance. The clinician must remain empathetic. The central conflict should be identified. Changes that advance the therapeutic process are not the province of conscious insight but the realm of unconscious procedural memory. Moment of clarity occur when a new set of implicit memories permit the therapy to progress leading to behavioral changes that expand the patient's range of procedural strategies (Kandal, 1999). The clinician is obliged to discourage dependency on the part of the patient (McCulloch, Ramesar & Peterson, 1998).

    The BATHE technique is a form of psychotherapy that is designed to be used by primary care clinicians and to be utilized in a fifteen minute visit (Figure 4.).

Figure 4. The BATHE Technique
Background: "What's going on in your life?"
Affective response: "How do you feel about that?"
Troubles: "What troubles you the most about that?"
Handling: "How are you handling that?"
Empathy: "That must be/have been very difficult?"

This technique may seem elementary but it does embody the essential elements discussed above. **B**ackground provides an opening for discussion and invites the addict to share concerns and stressors that may be sobriety threatening. Do not be tempted to ask the patient to tell you more. This may create confusion and break the therapeutic stride. **A**ffective response helps to prevent any possible miss interpretation of the patient's feelings. It will also give the clinician an idea of the patient's perceptions of the situation. Addicts need help labeling their feelings particularly if they were raised in an addictive home. **T**roubles help to identify the central concern, and provide focus and understanding for the clinician and the patient. A solution can be sought once the problem is identified. This line of questioning may provoke responses that trace their pain to childhood trauma. **H**andling sends the message that the professional respects the patient's method of dealing with challenges, promoting positive self-worth. It often helps the addict see a connection between their current behaviors and difficulties. The patient may wish to work with the clinician to develop new coping and problem solving techniques (Stuart & Lieberman, 1993). Addicts that are silent may appreciate the straightforward nature of these questions. Patients that are angry will benefit from empathic reflection and use this time to clarify their feelings and perceptions. The structure of this technique will help overly talkative individuals to focus. Patients can be redirected by asking, "Out of all these problems, what is most troublesome for you (McCulloch, Ramesar & Peterson, 1998)?"

The stories told by these people reflect their perception of reality. The clinician should respond in a way that reshapes the story to create more positive perceptions. Challenging their limits and educating the patient can do this. Absolutes need to be challenged. If the addict uses words such as: "always, never, can't or impossible", the clinician should respond with a phrase that can help the patient reshape their reality such as; "Have you ever…?" or "Has there ever been a time this worked for you?" Professionals need to believe in the power of the word "yet". This lets the addict know that someone believes in them. Patients that are empowered by this simple word will begin to look at life in a different light (Stuart & Lieberman, 1993).

There are several other **strategies** that can be employed to help addicts while using this technique. Focus on options when an individual presents with a life challenge. Addicts in crisis are not able to see options. This is an opportunity to teach problem solving skills. They have a choice when faced with a bad situation. They can leave it, they can change it, they can accept it or they can reframe it. They can also "choose not to choose". There are times when it is best not to act immediately. "Tincture of time" can allow some solutions to declare themselves, or make the problem someone else's. Help the addict to see the potential consequences of their choices. Help them gain perspective by asking them; what are the best thing and the worst thing that can happen with each option. Put the addict in control of their life. Make their strengths the focus of the interaction, not their weaknesses. Encourage **accountability**. Addicts must learn to accept responsibility for their behavior. Do not overwhelm the patient. Have them shoot for small victories. Teach the patient to "**live one day at a time**". The prospect of doing something new, such as remaining clean or changing behavior, is much easier to fathom if it is faced twenty-four hours at a time. The addict is able to avoid repeating behaviors driven by guilt by not living in the past, and they are able to avoid repeating behaviors driven by fear and pride by not living in the future (Stuart & Lieberman, 1993). Patients need to be instructed on the importance of changing "playmates, play grounds and play things". "Nothing changes, if nothing changes." The addict will continue to experience the same problems if they continue to place themselves in "sticky situations". Their spirituality can be enhanced by encouraging them to be positive and creative in all areas of their lives and by being of service to others.

There will be times when patients will become **angry or violent** during an interaction. Intoxication, metabolic derangement, psychiatric disorders and personality disorders heighten the risk of this occurring. These individuals may exhibit symptoms of motor restlessness and tension such as, pacing, drumming, and clenched fists or loud speech. The clinician must simultaneously help the patient and protest themselves and the staff. The situation needs to be controlled quickly. Do not react in a way that will escalate the situation. Honestly inventory your feelings and be aware of your part in the situation (Goldman,

1998). Make good eye contact and use a soft steady tone of voice to offer help. This will appeal to the patient's pride, which is trying to gain control. The next step is to follow the "**3 V's**". Allow the patient to **V**entilate their frustration, anger and fear. This acts as a catharsis. Then **V**alidate the patient's feelings and the situation. Agree that a problem exists and it is understandable that the individual feels the way they feel. Lastly, **V**enture hope that the situation can be dealt with and overcome (Jacobson, 1998).

There are several other psychotherapeutic modalities that may be offered to these patients. The basic principle of each of these techniques can be adapted for incorporation with the BATHE technique. **Cognitive-behavioral therapy** is based on the premise that learning processes play a critical role in the formation of maladaptive behavioral patterns. Addicts need to learn these patterns and adopt more acceptable substitutes. The professional will need to evaluate the addict's perceptions of the effects of their drug of choice or their behaviors, and the reasons for their substance use and behavior. Misconceptions should be challenged and alternatives should be explored (Fox & Weiner, 1982). Coping and social skills training are the core elements to CBT. Addicts are taught interpersonal skills to enhance relationships, cognitive-emotional coping skills for affect regulation, coping skills for "living life on life's terms" and coping skills to identify and deal with substance use cues. Addicts learn to refuse substances, give and receive positive and negative feedback, and conflict resolution (O'Leary & Monti, 2002).

Addicts tend to exhibit an assortment of self-defeating personality traits including, impulsivity, denial, rationalization, denial and self-pity. **Behavioral therapy** attempts to change the undesirable behavior by clearly demonstrating the desired behavior and rewarding steps taken toward the target behavior (Gallant, 1993). BT tries to help the individual gain three types of control. **Stimulus control** helps the patient change "playmates, playgrounds and play things" that were associated with drug use. They learn to spend their time in activities that are incompatible with substance use. **Urge control** involves recognizing and coping with emotions, cognition and sensations that occur with the impulse to use. **Social control** gets those close to the addict involved in helping the addict avoid substance use.

      Pastoral counseling may be in order if the patient has questions or issues regarding religion or spirituality. **Bibliotherapy** is another useful tool that can be incorporated into the management plan for the addicted patient. It simply involves assigned readings that can be discussed at follow up visits. Appendix 5 contains a list of readings that may be helpful.

References:

Fox S and Weiner H. (1982). Cognitive-behavioral therapy with substance abusers. *Social Casework; 63(9):* pp564-567.

Frank SH. (1993). Behavioral tools for the primary care doctor. *Family Practice; 10(1)*: pp23-33.

Gallant D. (1993). Amethystic agents and adjunct behavioral therapy and psychotherapy. *Alcoholism: Clinical and experimental research; 17(1)*: pp197-198.

Goldman B. (1998). Facing up to violent patients. *Emergency Medicine; 30(4)*: pp114-130.

Jacobson S. (1998). Streetwise in an emergency. *Emergency Medicine; 30(8)*: pp115-129.

Kandel, E. (1999). The biology and future of psychoanalysis: a new intellectual framework. *American Journal of Psychiatry; 156(4)*: pp505-524.

McCulloch J, Ramesar S and Peterson H. (1998). Psychotherapy in primary care: The BATHE technique. *American Family Physician; 57(9)*: pp2131- 2134.

Newburg AB and Newburg SK (1998). Incorporating stress management into clinical practice. *Hospital Physician; 34(6)*: pp52-58.

O'Leary TA and Monti PM. (2002). Cognitive-behavioral therapy for alcohol addiction. In: Hofmann SG, Tompson MC, Eds. *Treating chronic and severe mental disorders: A handbook of empirically supported interventions.* New York, NY: The Guilford Press. (pp234-57)

Sapolsky, P. (2003). Taming stress. *Scientific American; 289(3)*: pp86-95.

Seitz FC. (1997). Stress, Fear and illness (Tigers, caves and
    coping). In: Behavioral medicine made ridiculously
    simple. Miami: Med Master, Inc.
Stuart MR and Lieberman JA. (1993). *The fifteen minute hour:
    Applied psychotherapy for primary care physicians 2nd Ed.*
    Westport, Conn. Praeger.

Chapter 17
Spirituality

"Religion is for those that want to go to Heaven.
Spirituality is for those that have been to Hell."

-Anonymous

Spirituality is that which separates human beings from other creatures. In involves the values and beliefs that we choose to live by. It is the search for meaning and purpose; the deeper aspects of hope, love, connection, serenity, comfort and support. It is the ability to nurture the four natural relationships: relationship with self, family, community and a Higher Power. It is a connection with the world that surrounds us. Spirituality is relinquishing pride, guilt and fear in exchange for humility and faith, striving for a more selfless way of life and being of service to others. Spirituality is a behavioral response to another that happens as a consequence of giving to others, learning from others and relinquishing the Ego to a new Ego-ideal (French, 1993).

Overview:

Addicts express an array of common feelings and perceptions, including a sense of inferiority, unworthiness and a lack of connection. This is not surprising, as the addict has a diminished capacity for experiencing natural pleasure due to adaptations of the mesocorticolimbic system resulting from stress and substance exposure. They often relate this to having a spiritual void. Most addicts have experienced a great deal of psychological wounding because of their actions. Some addicts have the added burden of their troubled upbringing (Williams, 1998).

Spirituality can be conceptualized as the relationship between the **body, mind and emotions**. The disease of addiction affects all the above areas in a negative and destructive fashion. Over time this will create spiritual bankruptcy. Changes must be made to overcome this. The addict needs to act in a positive and creative way. When a problem develops the addict has to choose the positive and creative solution and avoid the negative and destructive path even if that seems to be the "easier, softer way". For the body they may eat healthier, stop using their drug of choice and begin to exercise. For the mind they may begin an education or explore new interests. For their emotions they may learn to express themselves, begin to pray and meditate, or attend a twelve-step group. The addict is "rewarded" with spiritual growth with each positive choice (Booth, 1995).

Enlightenment:

Addicts appear to be affected at **seven levels of consciousness** (Table 1.). The addict will progress though these levels as they obtain enlightenment and growth.

Table 1. The Seven Levels of Consciousness
Survival
Passion
Mind or ego
Acceptance
Understanding
Compassion
Unity conscious

At level one, addiction is a poison attacking the structures of the body. At the second level, addiction is painful and controlling, affecting emotional stability. At the third level, the stigma of addiction affects the mind and Ego, yielding a total absence of serenity. Most addicts become stuck in this level, never able to experience peace of mind. At the fourth level, the addict is at the "jumping of point". They are ambivalent about their problem but believe that recovery and personal growth are possible. At the fifth level, the disease of addiction is seen as a "gift". At the sixth level, the addict, now growing, compassionately helps others that are still suffering. At the seventh level, the addict feels fulfilled. This sense of purpose brings peace of mind and happiness (Whitfield, 1984).

Stages of Growth:

Dr. M. Scott Peck has identified **four stages of spiritual growth**. His work focuses on the religious aspect of spirituality, but may readily be applied to the recovery process. **Stage I** is the "chaotic/anti-social" stage. This stage corresponds to the developmental stage of a child less than 5 years of age. These people have an absence of spirituality. They feel no connection with anyone or anything. Like a young child, they have no principles and will lie, cheat and steal to get their way. They may pretend to be a loving person, but this is for self-serving motives. These individuals are examples of "self-will run riot" ruled by their Id. Their selfish acts create a life of chaos and turmoil.

Stage II is the "formal/institutional" stage. People at this stage begin to see the consequences of their actions and rely on an institution for direction and provide input to help the Superego gain influence and form a new Ego-ideal. This is usually a sudden advancement. The institution may be a prison, the military, church or a chemical dependency program. These individuals are very concrete and literal in their spiritual views and do not tolerate change well. For example, a person may be a model soldier, but may rapidly become a degenerate upon discharge from the military. These individuals will follow doctrine blindly without trying to explore any deeper meaning. They look at their Higher Power as an external force, not a force within themselves. They view their Higher Power as a punishing authority figure. With time, they begin to question doctrine and hypocrisy. This will cause them to "backslide" to stage I, or progress to stage III.

Stage III is the "skeptic/individual" stage. This stage corresponds to the developmental stage of adolescence; seeing how dogma conflicts with their developing Ego-ideal. These people question the "myth" and ritual of religion. They view the world in a very scientific way, looking for tangible evidence without reliance on blind faith. These individuals are not religious, yet they are not anti-social and act responsibly. They are capable of giving and receiving love and affection.

These people enter **stage IV** as they begin to see their inter-connectedness with the world around them and find psychic balance. This change is gradual and may never occur. They relish a mystery and actively seek out life's answers. They develop deep connections with others and view their Higher Power as existing everywhere including within them. This stage is the beginning of a personal spiritual path, developing a God of their understanding (Peck, 1993).

Recovery:

Let's discuss how this information **relates to recovery**. Patients that are actively using will be in stage I. They will be isolated from the four natural relationships, devoid of any sense of spiritual connection. Their lives are entrenched in chaos. These individuals may eventually develop a crisis that opens their eyes to the consequences of their drug abuse as their Ego defenses begin to collapse. This is the first step towards a spiritual awakening. These addicts will be open to suggestion and treatment for their addiction. They enter stage II at this point. They do very well in the structured environment of a treatment program. Some may appear as model patients while in rehabilitation, but relapse ('backslide") upon discharge when no longer in a controlled environment. Addicts that are in early recovery need to maintain structure. This is why it is suggested for them to keep a set schedule, attend ninety meetings in ninety days and to surround themselves with the fellowship of a 12-step program. These individuals need strict guidance and greatly benefit from the assistance of a **sponsor** or mentor that is familiar with the program and has a firm spiritual base. These people have a very black and white interpretation of the program and its materials. Their recovery is mostly based on fellowship and meetings. This is actually good at this stage as it helps to keep things simple and re-enforce structure. They will begin to experience some disillusionment over time. Their "pink cloud" will burst.

This is the beginning of stage III. It is important to have a good sponsor at this stage, as they are "at the jumping off point". These addicts can easily pull away from the program and isolate themselves. Their selfish motives will begin to drive their behaviors and they will slip back to stage I and be destined to relapse. With the right encouragement and handling they will continue on their journey. They should be instructed to have faith in the program and the process of spiritual growth, be encouraged to "dive" into the steps, and to provide service to others. During this time they continue to seek answers to their questions regarding life, spirituality and recovery. They develop a personal connection with their Higher Power and see the rewards of being positive and creative. They enter stage IV as they gain knowledge and apply it to their lives. Service will become an act of selflessness, only desiring to help another suffering person. There will be no ulterior motives. These acts of kindness create a sense of interconnectedness that gives the addict a purpose in life and true happiness.

Patients that have borderline personality disorder may be a challenge. They seem to be partially in each stage at the same time. Patients in stage one may be so manipulative that they try to give the impression of being at a higher stage of spiritual development in order to work the system for their favor. These people can be identified by their actions. They can "talk the talk, but don't walk the walk".

Spiritual Assessment:

It is helpful to **screen** for the patient's spiritual beliefs and practices prior to making spiritual recommendations. This helps to identify the current stage of spiritual development. The "**HOPE**" questions are a practical way to approach the spiritual assessment (Table 2.) (Anandarajah & Hight, 2001). This guide can be used to frame specific questions for each patient.

Table 2. The HOPE Questions for Spiritual Assessment
Sources of **H**ope, meaning, comfort, strength, peace, love and connection
Organized religion
Personal spirituality and **P**ractices
Effects on medical care and **E**nd-of-life issues

It is also important to identify any spiritual beliefs that may negatively affect health (Table 3.) (Koenig & Lewis, 2000). These **negative beliefs** may also present a barrier to growth and recovery and may be associated with a complicated grief reaction. These beliefs can be addressed with cognitive therapy or the patient can be referred to the appropriate clergy/spiritual advisor.

Table 3. Spiritual Beliefs Associated with Negative Outcomes
Viewing their Higher Power as punishing
Doubting their Higher Power's abilities
Passive religious deferral
Interpersonal religious discontent
Blaming demonic forces
Pleading for direct intercession
Expressing spiritual discontent

Spiritual issues can be dealt with by the clinician to greatly enhance the recovery process. The clergy best deals with religious matters. The clinician should be sensitive to the patient's beliefs and not try to impose their beliefs upon the patient.

Addiction Treatment:

Including a spiritual component to comprehensive **addiction treatment** may increase recovery rates and decrease relapse rates (Much, 1991; Jarusiewicz, 2000). An addict that is clean and sober without a spiritual program is not addressing their core problem, a lack of connection and a conflicted psyche. They become lonely and live with fear and guilt. Their behaviors are driven by self-centeredness. They become "restless, irritable and discontent" as they no longer have their drug of choice to numb their pain. They get to a point where they cannot take it. This is the moment that they chose between relapse, death or recovery. It is best to introduce the spiritual concepts of recovery in the first week of abstinence (Martin, Gass, Min & Allen, 2001). This catches the patient when they are in crisis and open to new concepts of change. Spiritual integration is not an easy process. Patients at lower stages of spiritual development may be threatened by concepts that relate to a more advanced stage. Spiritual development is classically obtained through a twelve-step program, such as Alcoholics Anonymous. **The twelve-steps** are a program of spiritual conversion and growth. The twelve-steps will be discussed in the next chapter. Spirituality in recovery is enhanced when the patient is honest, open-minded and willing (H.O.W.) (Sloan, 1999). The initial and most important step is that of surrender (Albers, 1994). This provides fertile ground for change and growth. The twelve-steps will ultimately yield several promises, which include "a new freedom and happiness". This is something foreign to the addict. Happiness is obtained through having a sense of purpose. This sense of purpose comes from helping others with addictions (King, 1995; Carroll, 1993).

The components of spirituality include meditation and prayer, following the 12-steps, surrendering control, practicing acceptance and forgiveness, developing mindfulness, by manifesting values, hope, and serenity. The patient can be aided on the spiritual journey with cognitive therapy. A therapist may use spirituality as a way to shape behavior; helping to strengthen the patient's adherence to spiritual principles (Martin & Booth, 1999). The goal of the spiritual platform is a capacity to make conscious choices, an ability to take growth-producing risks, an ability to develop healthy relationships, and a capacity to experience wonder and awe (Georgi, 1998). In essence, the clinician aids in changing the patient's negative perceptual filters, replacing them with positive perceptual filters while chipping away at Ego defenses. The addict can then see the world in a different light and begin to make changes that break their old patterns of behavior. Hence, "restoring them to sanity".

References:

French CV. (1993). Spirituality as a basis for recovery in alcoholics: A phenomenological approach. *Dissertation Abstracts International, 53(11)*: 5975B.

Williams GP. (1998). Adult children of alcoholics: Parental bonding, adult attachment, and spirituality. *Dissertation Abstracts International, 59(5)*: 2443B.

Booth L. (1995). New understanding of spirituality. *Journal of Chemical Dependency Treatment, 5(2)*: pp5-17.

Whitfield CL. (1984). *Alcoholism, other drug problems & spirituality: A transpersonal approach.* Baltimore, MD: The Resource Group. (p.142)

Peck MS. (1993). *Further along the road less traveled.* New York, New York: Simon & Schuster.

Anandarajah G and Hight E. (2001). Spirituality and medical practice: Using the HOPE questions as a practical tool for spiritual assessment. *American Family Physician; 63(1)*: pp81-89.

Koenig HG and Lewis G. (2000). Red flags – When faith does not heal. In: *The healing connection.* Nashville, Tn.: Word Publishing.

Much MJ. (1991). Effect of spirituality on recovery from alcoholism: A comparison between sober and relapsed alcoholics. *Dissertation Abstracts International, 52(9)*: 3185A.

Jarusiewicz B. (2000). Spirituality and addiction: Relationship to recovery and relapse. *Alcoholism Treatment Quarterly, 18(4):* pp99-110.

Martin C, Gass CA, Min D and Allen AT. (2001). Spirituality in substance abuse detoxification treatment. *Journal of Addictive Diseases, 20(2)*: p158.

Sloan HP. (1999). God imagery and emergent spirituality in early recovery from chemical dependency: Ana-Maria Rizzuto and the Alcoholics Anonymous Twelve-Steps. *Dissertation Abstracts International, 60(6)*: 2085A.

Albers RH. (1994). Spirituality and surrender: A theological analysis of Tiebout's theory for Ministry to the alcoholic. *Journal of Ministry in Addiction and Recovery, 1(2)*: pp47-69.

King, DJ. (1995). Applied spirituality: Expressing love and service. *Journal of Chemical Dependency Treatment, 5(2)*: pp117-134.

Carroll, S. (1993). Spirituality and purpose in life in alcoholism recovery. *Journal of Studies on Alcohol, 54(3)*: pp297-301.

Martin JE and Booth J. (1999). Behavioral approaches to enhance spirituality. In: Miller WR, Ed., *Integrating Spirituality into Treatment: Resources for Practitioners*. Washington, DC: American Psychological Association. (pp161-175)

Georgi JM. (1998). Spiritual platform: Spirituality and psychotherapy in addiction medicine. *North Carolina Medical Journal, 59(3)*: pp168-171.

Chapter 18
Twelve-step Programs
"If you surrendered to the air, you could ride it."
-Toni Morrison

The first twelve-step program was **Alcoholics Anonymous (A.A.)**. It was founded on June 10, 1935 with a chance meeting of a New York stock speculator and an Akron Ohio physician. Bill Wilson was a businessman that struggled with alcoholism throughout most of his adult life. He had been institutionalized several times because of his addiction. He met Dr. William D. Silkworth during one of these hospitalizations. Dr. Silkworth told Bill about his theory that alcoholism was a disease and not a moral flaw. Dr. Silkworth felt that alcoholics have a type of "allergy" to alcohol. The first drink triggers a "phenomena of craving" that creates an obsession to continue drinking with no regard for the potential consequences. Bill thought this knowledge would be enough to keep him sober, but it wasn't. He returned to his prior path in just a few weeks. He couldn't understand what was happening and he felt hopeless.

An old alcoholic friend, named Ebby visited Bill. Ebby seemed different to Bill. He was neat and clean. He had an air of peace surrounding him. Ebby told Bill of how, three months prior, he was facing committal to a psychiatric institution for chronic alcoholism. A group of strangers asked the judge if they could have an opportunity to work with him. These people were from a Christian service organization called the Oxford Group. They instructed Ebby on their basic tenets which included "cleaning house", living a principle centered life, and service to others. Ebby told Bill of his experience with the Oxford Group and how he was able to apply their methods to remain sober. This was the second piece of the puzzle for Bill. Once again, Bill found himself in the hospital. This is where he had a spiritual awakening. He realized that it wasn't the last drink that got him drunk, it was the first. He also knew that he was going to have to reach out to other alcoholics if he was going to remain sober himself (Anonymous, 1984).

Bill worked very closely with the Oxford Group doing everything he could for the alcoholic that was still suffering. None of his prospects remained sober. However, Bill did remain sober. While in Akron on business, Bill struggled with the desire to drink. He knew that he would need to reach out to another alcoholic if he were to maintain his sobriety. He contacted the local Oxford Group. They gave him the name of a prospect that agreed to meet with him for fifteen minutes. This man was Dr. Robert Smith. Bill approached Dr. Bob differently than he had approached his other prospects. He began by telling Bob that he didn't come to help him get sober. Bill said that he was there to stay sober himself. He then tried to relate to Bob by telling his drinking history. Bill then told Bob of Dr. Silkworth's theory and of the Oxford Group's philosophies. Their conversation lasted several hours and was the beginning of A.A. They began to work diligently to help other alcoholics forming a fledgling group in Akron. Together, they developed the concepts of recovery that would become the twelve-steps (Anonymous, 1984).

This organization demonstrated miraculous growth over the years and has served as a prototype for many other twelve-step organizations. The growth and survival of this organization is attributed to the twelve-traditions of the organization (see Appendix 3). Al-anon is a direct spin off of A.A. It was formed in Canada in the early 1950s to help the loved ones of those inflicted with an addiction. This group views alcoholism as a family disease and uses the twelve-steps to help the family recover. Narcotics Anonymous was founded in 1953. They originated in California. This was a period in our nation's history that was marked by rebellion and escalating narcotic use. Addicts initially went to A.A. to learn a new way of life, but this conflicted with A.A.'s singleness of purpose. They discovered that they had certain issues that they didn't feel comfortable sharing in A.A. and that a group of their own design would be more helpful (Anonymous, 1987). Appendix 4 contains a list of several twelve-step organizations and how to contact them.

Twelve-step organizations are about **integrity**. They not only instruct the addict to "live life on life's" terms by "doing the next right thing", these programs help the addict to integrate or achieve wholeness. They use the twelve-steps to become open to the conflicting forces, ideas and stresses of their past and present situations. They learn to integrate their mind, emotions and bodies to become accountable and to achieve spiritual enlightenment; bringing the Id, Superego and Ego into balance. They will ultimately re-integrate with their family, society and Higher Power.

There are many ways that twelve-step programs help addicts to become whole. They are programs of spiritual conversion, leading the individual toward stage IV spiritual growth. This conversion will help to transform fear into faith, and pride and self-pity into humility. They place reliance on a Higher Power, without being associated with any specific religion. The spiritual principles are compatible with Christian, Jewish, Muslim, and Buddhist beliefs, as well as atheism. They are psychological programs, using the twelve-steps as a tool to examine past experiences to identify aberrant behaviors, the motivation behind the behaviors and possible alternative behaviors; bringing unconscious acts and defense mechanisms to consciousness. Programs such as A.A. use slogans in a repetitive fashion to aid recall in early recovery (See Appendix 1).

The newly recovering individual is encouraged to get a **sponsor**. The sponsor serves as a mentor and a lay therapist. The sponsor guides the individual through the steps and helps the addict to live responsibly with out using a chemical as an escape from reality. These are also programs of community. The fellowship of the program is based on the individuals facing a common crisis and having a common bond. This helps the addict to form healthy relationships and emerge from isolation (Peck, 1993).

We will now take a more detailed look at each of the twelve-steps of Alcoholics Anonymous. This overview will be quite basic and will be directed toward the alcoholic. It should be noted that the words alcoholic or alcohol could easily be substituted by words such as drugs, sex, gambling and food, and these steps would be just as applicable.

Step 1: We admitted we were powerless over alcohol – that our lives had become unmanageable. This is the surrender step and the only step that must be done 100%. Any less and the person will be doomed to relapse. This step deals with acceptance of the disease of addiction; understanding that alcohol and other mind altering substances can not ever be safely ingested. That addiction is a physical illness leading the affected individual toward compulsive enslavement to a substance. The search for and use of alcohol drove the alcoholic's life. The primary goal of motivational interviewing is to help those affected with this disease take the first step (Anonymous, 1994).

Step 2: Came to believe that a Power greater than ourselves could restore us to sanity. This step deals with the behavioral changes that occur with addiction. The individual is driven by a self-centered need to fulfill their desires. They will manipulate anyone or anything to reach their selfish goals, each time creating more adverse consequences and chaos. **Insanity** is defined as repeating the same behaviors and actions, while expecting different results. The alcoholic's behavior is certainly insane regarding substance use. The person new to recovery will be overwhelmed by such a drastic change. They will need the help of a Power greater than themselves. Initially this power may simply be the twelve-step program as it is a higher power with a proven track record. The individual will develop their own concept of God as they grow spiritually and the fog clears (Anonymous, 1994).

Step 3: Made a decision to turn our will and our lives over to the care of God, as we understood Him. This step involves a decision to proceed with the rest of the steps, using **G**ood **O**rderly **D**irection to guide the thoughts (will) and actions (life) of the addict. This is a tremendous commitment that acknowledges the spiritual nature of recovery. This step may be challenging to some individuals as their concept of God may be based on their parental relationship.

Step 4: Made a searching and fearless moral inventory of ourselves. This is a thorough and honest behavioral analysis. A problem can not be corrected unless it is first identified. This is the first of the "house cleaning" steps.

Human beings are endowed with **three natural instincts**. These instincts encompass the Id. Each of these instincts serves a role in the survival of our race. The first is the sex instinct, which insures reproduction and the continuation of the species. The second is the social instinct, which guides us to form a community and function as a society with interdependence amongst its members. The final instinct is for security. This instinct has two parts, material (financial) security, which drives us to seek food and shelter, and emotional security, which guides us toward the search for peace and happiness. Each of these instincts may exceed their intended function, blindly driving us toward a self-centered existence. If balance is lost and we become driven by one instinct, the other areas of our life will suffer. For example, if an individual is driven primarily by their instinct for material security they may act out of greed. They may become willing to lie, cheat and steal in order to satisfy their appetite. These behaviors will arouse anger, jealousy and revenge in others, and guilt within oneself. This leads to poor relationships and isolation. It is easy to see how both under or over focus in each of these instincts can breed a multitude of character defects and result in tumultuous relationships and a chaotic life (Wilson, 1988).

The Big Book of Alcoholics Anonymous asks the member to list ALL of their resentments (people, institutions and principles). Write down why the addict is resentful in each instance. Finally the addict must look at his or her own part in each situation. Seeing how each of the three instincts may have been threatened and how pride, self-pity and fear fueled their response. Anger and resentment are luxuries the addict can not afford, as these emotions will surely lead to relapse. Next, it is suggested to list all their fears and the associated situations. Then try to correlate each fear with a distortion of instinct and how it was acted upon. Fear is usually associated with the acquisition or the loss of something from the three instincts. This causes the individual to make unrealistic demands on one-self and others, and teaches the person to never be satisfied. Ego defense mechanisms justify the excesses of behavior. The final part of this step is a review of past relationships. Listing past sexual conduct, what went wrong and how selfish behavior was driven by dysfunctional instincts (Anonymous, 1976).

This exercise is a form of behavioral therapy. The alcoholic is able to examine his or her behavior, identify any defects of character and identify the underlying motivation behind the aberrant behavior. Some patients will have a tremendous amount of fear associated with performing this step. There may be a great deal of shame and guilt due to past actions. These feelings commonly lead to procrastination. Not performing this step in a timely fashion, to the best of the alcoholic's ability for the given time, is a recipe for relapse.

Step 5: Admitted to God, to ourselves, and to another human being the exact nature of our wrongs. This step is the step that opens the doors toward a spiritual path. **Narcissism** is the principle precursor of psycho-spiritual illness. People with addictions are masters of rationalization and justification. By sharing step 4 with another individual, the alcoholic is able to gain insights from someone whose vision is not clouded by pride, self-pity and fear. This step is usually taken with the alcoholic's sponsor or a member of the clergy. This outside party will aid in uncovering the motives behind prior acts, to see through the alcoholic's narcissism and challenge it. The alcoholic will be able to see their past for what it is, the accumulated actions and consequences of a conflicted psyche. They will be able to see that they are no worse and no better than anyone else. If this step is done with total honesty, this will yield the first spark of true **humility**. They will become less aware of themselves and more aware of others (Wilson, 1988).

Step 6: Were entirely ready to have God remove all these defects of character.

Step 7: Humbly asked Him to remove our shortcomings. These steps are usually performed at or near the same time. The alcoholic may go through a period of grieving once they have identified their part in past conflicts, have identified their fears and the underlying factors, and have identified how their relationships were dysfunctional. The alcoholic can progress toward change once the reality of the past is accepted. This action will bring on a type of moral empowerment; helping them to integrate their past with their new ideals. These changes can be more overwhelming than the prospect of not drinking or using. These defects of character are the dysfunctional behaviors that helped the Ego survive while in active addiction. Therefore, it is best to not attempt this change alone. Reliance must be placed on a Higher Power such as, the fellowship, the twelve-steps, good orderly direction or God (Anonymous, 1994).

Step 8: Made a list of all persons we had harmed, and became willing to make amends to them all. This step involves further housecleaning. The addict uses the lists made in step 4 and the knowledge from step 5 to compile a list of individuals that have been harmed because of their selfish behaviors. The alcoholic looks at the part they played in each of their resentments and dysfunctional relationships. The addict examines each of these events and issues, and becomes **accountable** for their actions (Wilson, 1988).

Step 9: Made direct amends to such people wherever possible, except when to do so would injure them or others. With accountability comes responsibility. The addict has a responsibility to not only apologize but to set right what went wrong. With family, this will mean leading a sober principle centered life. With creditors, this will mean paying debts. The key to this step is **restitution**, not another empty apology. The exception to doing this is when the direct amends would lead to injuring another. This can occur when the other individual is not aware of the infraction, such as infidelity, or with confession of a crime that would implicate others. The addict cannot obtain peace of mind at the expense of another person's serenity (Wilson, 1988).

This is a pivotal step for the person in recovery. The goal of recovery is not mere abstinence from substance abuse; it is developing a new way of living in reality. This lofty goal is exemplified by the "Ninth Step Promises" that are said to occur once the wreckage of the past has been cleared. The following is an exert from *The Big Book of Alcoholics Anonymous*.

> "If we are painstaking about this phase of our development, we will be amazed before we are half way through. We are going to know a new freedom and a new happiness. We will not regret the past nor wish to shut the door on it. We will comprehend the word serenity and we will know peace. No matter how far down the scale we have gone, we will see how our experience can benefit others. That feeling of uselessness and self-pity will disappear. We will lose interest in selfish things and gain interest in our fellows. Self-seeking will slip away. Our whole attitude and outlook upon life will change. Fear of people and of economic insecurity will leave us. We will intuitively know how to handle situations that used to baffle us. We will suddenly realize that God is doing for us what we could not do for ourselves."
> "Are these extravagant promises? We think not. They are being fulfilled among us—sometimes quickly, sometimes slowly. They will always materialize if we work for them (Anonymous, 1976)."

Step 10: Continued to take personal inventory and when we were wrong promptly admitted it. This is the **maintenance** step. The prior steps looked at the past and cleaned up the wreckage. This step looks at the alcoholic's daily progress. Where were old self-seeking behaviors replaced with new virtuous behaviors? Where did the old behaviors resurface and create conflict. The alcoholic must admit fault when old behaviors are exhibited. If they readily make amends there will be only a limited risk of developing guilt, remorse and other forms of self-pity. The alcoholic will be able to avoid breading new resentments. This process should not be a form of self-praise or self-punishment, it should be an educational exploration with the intent of nurturing spiritual growth (Wilson, 1988).

Step 11: Sought through prayer and meditation to improve our conscious contact with God as we understood Him, praying only for knowledge of His will for us and the power to carry that out. With this step, the alcoholic is acknowledging that they cannot take the credit for the successes of their new life. True humility calls for "giving the credit where credit is do". This means turning to their Higher Power with gratitude. It also means being accountable and taking on the responsibility for the bad things that have happened as a result of their actions. Daily practice of prayer and meditation help to keep the alcoholic on the right track. This practice aids in relaxation, replenishing the alcoholic's mental, physical and spiritual energies. Simply put, God's will is for each individual to love his fellow man and for each alcoholic not to drink. It is not to micromanage the finer points of an individual's life (Anonymous, 1994).

Step 12: Having had a spiritual awakening as a result of these steps, we tried to carry this message to alcoholics, and to practice these principles in all our affairs. By working the steps the alcoholic will realize that he or she is not an isolated entity; that each individual is connected to the next and that we are all inter-connected with the world around us. Each decision made and action taken not only affects the individual, but also affects those around them. The alcoholic will begin to check his or her motives before acting and in turn will cease to react selfishly. When reviewing the successes of their life, the alcoholic will experience humble gratitude, not pride and grandiosity. To maintain this new way of life it becomes imperative for the alcoholic to "share their experience, strength and hope" with the alcoholic that still suffers. They learn that the rewards of **service** to others are much greater than any imagined. One of the great paradoxes of spirituality is that to keep what has been gained; it must be given away (Anonymous, 1976).

Twelve-step program attendance has demonstrated outcomes that are equal to cognitive behavioral therapy (Ouimette, Finney & Moos, 1997). Patients honestly working a twelve-step program will present on follow up with a new level of **maturity**. They will begin to see meeting life's demands as an opportunity for growth, no longer complaining when life does not meet their expectations. Patients that are not working a good program will present with the warning signs of the process of **relapse**. The individual will begin to have "mental binges". This is when they revert back to self-centered behaviors. They feel victimized. They try to control their external environment. They begin to think that certain rules should not apply in their case; self- centeredness and self-seeking result in the classic symptoms of being "restless, irritable and discontent". The patient may then progress towards "spiritual blackouts" as they see the world through negative perceptual filters. They will withdrawal from the fellowship, their family and society in general. They lose any sense of connectedness, and they will become the center of their universe. They will no longer have the ability to cope and "face life on life's terms". These patients will be at a critical juncture. Their despair will lead them to the **crossroads** of insanity, suicide or relapse.

What can a primary care physician do to help patients in twelve-step programs? Taking an interest in your patient's program helps a great deal. Record the patient's sobriety date in their chart and give them praise for anniversaries; celebrated at 1 month, 3 months, 6 months, 9 months, 1 year and then annually. When the patient comes in for any chief complaint, ask them what step they are working on and how often they speak with their sponsor. Patients that are progressing well with their program will be actively working the steps even after years of sobriety. These patients will also have regular contact with their sponsor. Try to identify any barriers to recovery if the patient does not seem to be complying with the suggestions of the program. Recommend that they contact their sponsor daily or recommend that they get a sponsor if they do not have one. Suggest attending ninety meetings in ninety days if the addict has recently relapsed or has recently been discharged from a treatment center. It may be helpful for patients to attend twelve-step facilitated therapy if they are having problems grasping the program or have had repeated relapses (Gossop, Stewart & Marden, 2008). Refer them to a clergyman of their particular faith if the individual is having problems with their concept of God. It may be best to refer the patient back to their sponsor if this challenge is because of a prior religious (dogmatic) conflict. The steps are also a useful way to examine the behavior of patients when performing the BATHE technique (See Chapter 16).

References:

Anonymous. (1976). *Alcoholics Anonymous: The story of how many thousands of men and women have recovered from alcoholism, 3rd edition.* New York, New York: Alcoholics Anonymous World Services, Inc.

Anonymous (1984). *Pass it on: The story of Bill Wilson and how the A.A. message reached the world.* New York, New York: Alcoholics Anonymous World Services , Inc.

Anonymous (1987). *Narcotics Anonymous, 4th edition.* Van Nuys, California: World Services Office, Inc.,

Anonymous. (1994). *The little red book.* Center City, Minnesota: Hazelden information and education services.

Gossop, M., Stewart, D. and Marsden, J. (2008). Attendence at Narcotics Anonymous and Alcoholics Anonymous meetings, frequency of attendance and substance use outcomes after residential treatment for drug dependence: a 5-year follow-up study. *Addiction; 103(1)*: pp119-125.

Ouimette, P., Finney, J. and Moos, R. (1997). Twelve-step and cognitive-behavioral treatment for substance abuse a comparison of treatment effectiveness. *Journal of Consulting and Clinical Psychology; 65(2)*: pp230-240.

Peck MS. (1993). *Further along the road less traveled: The unending journey toward spiritual growth.* New York, New York: Simon and Schuster.

Wilson W. (1988). *The twelve steps and twelve traditions.* New York, New York: Alcoholics Anonymous World Services , Inc.

Chapter 19
Treatment Programs
"People must help one another; it is nature's law."
-Jean De La Fontaine

Many addicts are able to find recovery without being admitted to a formal treatment program, but this is difficult for the addict and they must be highly motivated. Addicts exhibit behaviors that help them to survive while using their drug of choice. These survival skills are self-centered and self-seeking by nature and are not compatible with living a sober life. These behaviors breed chaos, resentment and fear, all of which are sure to lead the addict, back down the road of addiction. The disease of addiction is a complex dysfunction of the mind, body and spirit and some addicts are best managed in a formal treatment setting.

Managed Care:
Managed care cuts have made it more difficult to place patients into inpatient rehabilitation programs. These organizations have unrealistic expectations and equate addiction as simply using drugs or alcohol, and recovery as abstinence. They follow an acute care model and expect outcomes similar to the outcomes of acute illnesses (McLellan, McKay, Forman, Cacciola & Kemp, 2005). The disease of addiction is complex and this misunderstanding has been a barrier for people seeking help. Addiction treatment appears to be as effective as treatment of other chronic diseases. Drug addiction treatment is cost effective.

It has been estimated that for every dollar spent on addiction treatment, between four and seven dollars are saved in reduced crime, theft and judicial costs alone. This does not take into account the economic benefits of returning an addict to the work force or the reduced cost of health care. The ratio is over 12:1 when these areas are factored into the equation.

Overview of Treatment:

Several principles have been identified that assist in the selection of the most **effective addiction treatment** setting. No single treatment center is right for everyone. The treatment setting should have services that can accommodate the addict's individual needs. This may include specialized psychological counseling or programs to improve life skills. Treatment needs to be readily accessible as to not miss a window of opportunity and give the patient time to back out. The addict's treatment plan must be assessed and modified on a continual basis to adapt to their changing requirements. Strategies should be employed to keep the individual engaged in treatment, avoiding premature departure.

Research has indicated that most patients reach the threshold of significant improvement at **ninety days**, but longer periods of time can yield further advances.

Counseling and behavioral therapy are critical for these patients. Certain addicts may require medications that aid in quelling cravings and psychiatric symptoms. These institutions should offer resources that help the addict address their psychiatric problems. Patients in treatment need to be monitored for substance use. The needs of **women** in addiction treatment differ from the needs of men. Barriers to women receiving treatment are removed when these needs are met. These needs include child care, prenatal care programs that address female-focused topics, programs dealing with abuse, and programs addressing relationships. Some women may benefit from women only programs (Ashley, Marsden & Brady, 2003). Treatment programs should provide assessment and monitoring of the physical complications of addiction, such as hepatitis, HIV/AIDS and tuberculosis.

Outpatient verses Residential:

Highly motivated addicts with extensive social supports may do well in an **outpatient** drug-free treatment program. These programs vary greatly in services offered. They tend to be cheaper than inpatient or residential programs. Low-intensity programs may only provide drug education, while intensive outpatient programs offer a wide range of services. They often provide individual and group counseling, behavioral therapy, education and psychiatric treatment. Some studies have demonstrated that intensive outpatient programs have similar social and drug use outcomes as more costly inpatient programs (Belcnko, Patapis & French, 2005).

The Matrix Model is a multimodality intensive outpatient program that was developed to treat cocaine addicts in the 1980s with great success. The program as been further tailored to meet the needs of addicts addicted to other stimulants such as methamphetamine. The program lasts 16 weeks and consists of structured group sessions targeting relapse prevention. Patients also meet with a therapist on an individual basis. There is a 12-week family and patient education component. Patients are expected to undergo weekly drug testing and attend twelve-step meetings (Rawson, Shoptaw, Obert, McCann, Hassson, Marinelli-Casey, Brethen & Ling, 1995).

Short-term residential programs provide brief intensive inpatient therapy in a hospital setting. These programs traditionally use a twelve-step approach. They typically last twenty-eight days and involve counseling, behavioral therapy, and education. Life skills and psychological issues can also be addressed.

Long-term residential programs provide 24-hour care in a non-hospital setting. Most centers use the "therapeutic community" as a treatment model. The therapeutic community is a simulated structured social environment that helps the addict re-integrate into society. Addiction is viewed in the context of their social and psychological issues. Therapy focuses on developing interpersonal communication, accountability, and sociability. Programs are highly structured and tend to be confrontational. Activities are geared toward the patient examining their damaging belief systems, their behaviors and their self-conceptions. These programs are very comprehensive, lasting as long as twelve-months, and involve a wide range of services. The **criminal justice system** offers programs to offenders. These programs are similar to the other programs and participants are heavily monitored for substance use.

References:

Ashley, O., Marsden, M. and Brady, T. (2003). Effectiveness of substance abuse treatment programming for women: a review. *The American Journal of Drug and Alcohol Abuse: 29(1)*: pp19-53.

Belenko, S., Patapis, N., & French, M. T. (2005). *Economic benefits of drug treatment: A critical review of the evidence for policy makers.* Philadelphia: Treatment Research Institute, University of Pennsylvania.

McLellan, A., McKay, J., Forman, R., Cacciola, J. and Kemp, J. (2005). Reconsidering the evaluation of addiction treatment: from a retrospective follow-up to concurrent recovery monitoring. *Addiction; 100(4)*: pp447-458.

Rawson, R., Shoptaw, S., Obert, J., McCann, M., Hassson, A., Marinelli-Casey, P. Brethen, P. and Ling, W. (1995). An intensive outpatient approach for cocaine abuse treatment: The Matrix model. *Journal of Substance Abuse Treatment, 12: 117-127.*

Appendix 1: Recovery Slogans

One day at a time.

First things first.

Progress not perfection.

Turn it over.

HALT (Don't get too hungry, angry, lonely, tired)

Too much analyzing, leads to paralyzing.

FEAR (False Evidence Appearing Real)

FEAR (Face Everything And Recover)

KISS (Keep It Simple Stupid)

Thy will be done, not mine!

Identify, don't compare.

Don't analyze, utilize!

Don't should on yourself.

When I'm in my own head, I'm in a bad neighborhood.

Take what you want and leave the rest.

Develop an attitude of gratitude.

You're only as sick as your secrets!

HOW? (Honesty, Open-mindedness, Willingness)

Let go and let God!

Good Orderly Direction

Feelings aren't always facts.

This too shall pass!

Don't give up before the Miracle.

Stinkin' thinkin' leads to drinkin'!

SIN (Self-Imposed Nonsense)

ASAP (Always Say A Prayer)

Appendix 2: The Twelve-steps Of Alcoholics Anonymous ®

1. We admitted we were powerless over alcohol, that our lives had become unmanageable.

2. Came to believe that a Power greater than ourselves could restore us to sanity.

3. Made a decision to turn our will and our lives over to the care of God <u>as we understood Him.</u>

4. Made a searching and fearless moral inventory of ourselves.

5. Admitted to God, to ourselves, and to another human being the exact nature of our wrongs.

6. Were entirely ready to have God remove all these defects of character.

7. Humbly asked Him to remove our shortcomings.

8. Made a list of all persons we had harmed, and became willing to make amends to the all.

9. Made direct amends to such people wherever possible, except when to do so would injure them or others.

10. Continued to take personal inventory and when we were wrong promptly admitted it.

11. Sought through prayer and meditation to improve our conscious contact with God <u>as we understood Him,</u> praying only for knowledge of his will for us and the power to carry that out.

12. Having had a spiritual awakening as the result of these steps, we tried to carry this message to alcoholics, and to practice these principles in all our affairs.

Appendix 3: The Twelve-traditions of Alcoholics Anonymous ®

1. Our common welfare should come first; personal recovery depends on A.A. unity.

2. For our group purpose there is but one ultimate authority—a loving God as He may express Himself in our group conscience. Our leaders are but trusted servants; they do not govern.

3. The only requirement for A.A. membership is a desire to stop drinking.

4. Each group should be autonomous except in matters affecting other groups or A.A. as a whole.

5. Each group has but one primary purpose—to carry its message to the alcoholic who still suffers.

6. An A.A. group ought never endorse, finance, or lend the A.A. name to any related facility or outside enterprise, lest problems of money, property, and prestige divert us from our primary purpose.

7. Every A.A. group ought to be fully self-supporting, declining outside contributions.

8. Alcoholics Anonymous should remain forever nonprofessional, but our service centers may employ special workers.

9. A.A., as such, ought never be organized; but we may create service boards or committees directly responsible to those they serve.

10. Alcoholics Anonymous has no opinion on outside issues; hence the A.A. name ought never be drawn into public controversy.

11. Our public relations policy is based on attraction rather than promotion; we need always maintain personal anonymity at the level of press, radio, and films.

12. Anonymity is the spiritual foundation of all our traditions, ever reminding us to place principles before personalities.

Appendix 4: Recovery Resources

Adult Children of Alcoholics
World Services Office
P.O. Box 3216
Torrance, Ca 90510
(310) 534-1815
www.adultchildren.org

Al-Anon/Alateen
World Service Office
1600 Corporate Landing Parkway
Virginia Beach, Va 23454-5617
www.al-anon.alateen.org

Alcoholics Anonymous
Grand Central Station
P.O. Box 459
New York, NY 10163
www.alcoholics-anonymous.org

American Society of Addiction Medicine
4601 North Park Avenue
Arcade Suite 101
Chevy Chase, Md 20815
(301) 656-3920
www.asam.org

Cocaine Anonymous
World Service Office
3740 Overland Avenue
Los Angeles, Ca 90034
(310) 559-5833
www.ca.org

Dual Recovery Anonymous
World Services Central Office
P.O. Box 8107
Praire Village, Ks 66208
(877) 883-2332
http://draonline.org

Gamblers Anonymous
International Service Office
P.O. Box 17173
Los Angeles, Ca 90017
(213) 386-8789
www.gamblersanonymous.org

Narcotics Anonymous
World Services Office
P.O. Box 9999
Van Nuys, Ca 91409
(818) 773-9999
www.na.org

National Institute of Alcohol Abuse and Alcoholism
www.niaaa.nih.gov

National Institute of Drug Abuse
www.nida.nih.gov

Overeaters Anonymous
World Services Office
P.O. Box 44020
Rio Rancho, NM 87174-4020
www.oa.org

Sex Addicts Anonymous
International Service Office
P.O. Box 70949
Houston, Tx 77270
(800) 477-8191
www.sexaa.org

Sexaholics Anonymous
International Central Office
P.O. Box 3565
Brentwood, Tn 37024
(614) 370-6062
www.sa.org

Index

www.ingramcontent.com/pod-product-compliance
Lightning Source LLC
Chambersburg PA
CBHW051450170526
45166CB00001B/188